In *Depression in New Mothers*, Vol II, Kathleen Kendall-Tackett provides a clear clinical context for the necessity of effective screening and assessment as the critical link to promoting successful treatment outcomes. She identifies the wide range of screening tools, their benefits and drawbacks, and current evidence-based treatments beyond just a pharmacological approach. This text is an invaluable roadmap for best practices in decision-making for the field of maternal mental health.

—**Diana L. Barnes**, *PsyD PMH-C, private practice,*
perinatal mental health, San Diego

This book comprehensively overviews screening and treatment options for a woman experiencing perinatal mental health conditions. It covers evidenced-based complementary, alternative, and integrative therapies as well. An amazing overview of psychotherapy as a treatment and a review of medication options. A highly recommended informative book for practitioners in the field of perinatal mental health.

—**Birdie Gunyon Meyer**, *RN, MA, PMH-C, Certification and*
Training Director, Postpartum Support International

Depression in New Mothers, Volume 2

This fourth edition of *Depression in New Mothers, Volume 2: Screening, Assessment, and Treatment Alternatives* provides a comprehensive and evidence-based approach to understanding the assessment for treatment and treatment of postpartum depression.

Depression, anxiety, and posttraumatic stress disorder are common complications of childbirth that result in adverse health outcomes for both mother and child. It is vital, therefore, that health professionals be ready to help women with these conditions in the perinatal period. Written by a psychologist and board-certified lactation consultant, this fourth edition is greatly expanded and available as two complementary volumes. Focusing on causes and consequences of poor perinatal mental health and its treatment. It can also be used by community organizations that want to support new mothers, screen for possible depression, discuss treatment options, and refer them to appropriate care. This volume integrates current international research and includes chapters on:

- Choosing an assessment scale to measure depression and co-occurring conditions
- Developing a treatment plan
- Supporting new mothers and families through community interventions
- Using complementary and integrative therapies
- Providing evidence-based psychotherapy
- Using antidepressants

Depression in New Mothers, Volume 2 (4th Edition) includes case illustrations throughout and retains its focus on moving research into practice. It is an essential resource for all healthcare practitioners working with mothers in the perinatal period, including mental health providers, nurses, midwives, doctors, lactation consultants, and peer supporters.

Kathleen A. Kendall-Tackett is a health psychologist and international board–certified lactation consultant (IBCLC). Dr. Kendall-Tackett is Editor-in-Chief of the journal *Psychological Trauma*. She is a fellow of the American Psychological Association in Health and Trauma Psychology, the past president of the APA Division of Trauma Psychology, and a member of Postpartum Support International's President's Advisory Council. Dr. Kendall-Tackett has published over 500 articles on women's health, breastfeeding, depression, trauma, and health psychology. This is her 42nd book.

Depression in New Mothers, Volume 2

Screening, Assessment, and Treatment Alternatives

Fourth Edition

Kathleen A. Kendall-Tackett

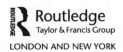
Routledge
Taylor & Francis Group

LONDON AND NEW YORK

Designed cover image: Getty Images

Fourth edition published 2024
by Routledge
4 Park Square, Milton Park, Abingdon, Oxon, OX14 4RN

and by Routledge
605 Third Avenue, New York, NY 10158

Routledge is an imprint of the Taylor & Francis Group, an informa business

© 2024 Kathleen A. Kendall-Tackett

First edition published by Routledge 2005
Second edition published by Routledge 2009
Third edition published by Routledge 2016

British Library Cataloguing-in-Publication Data
A catalogue record for this book is available from the British Library

Library of Congress Cataloging-in-Publication Data
Names: Kendall-Tackett, Kathleen A., author.
Title: Depression in new mothers / Kathleen A. Kendall-Tackett.
Description: Fourth edition. | Milton Park, Abingdon, Oxon ; New York, NY :
    Routledge, 2024. | Includes bibliographical references and index. |
    Contents: Volume 1. Causes, consequences, and risk factors —
Identifiers: LCCN 2023024798 | ISBN 9781032532776 (volume 1; hardback) |
    ISBN 9781032532752 (volume 1; paperback) | ISBN 9781003411246 (volume 1;
    ebook)
Subjects: LCSH: Postpartum depression.
Classification: LCC RG852 .K448 2024 | DDC 618.7/6—dc23/eng/20230717
LC record available at https://lccn.loc.gov/2023024798

ISBN: 978-1-032-52077-3 (hbk)
ISBN: 978-1-032-52074-2 (pbk)
ISBN: 978-1-003-40509-2 (ebk)

DOI: 10.4324/9781003405092

Typeset in Sabon
by Apex CoVantage, LLC

Contents

Foreword   *xiii*
DIANE SANFORD

Preface   *xv*

SECTION I
Screening for Depression and CoMorbid Conditions   1

1 Screening: Rationale and Barriers   3

Why Screening Is Helpful 3
Barriers to Screening 4
Screening in Pediatric Settings 5
   Barriers to Screening 6
Screening in Obstetric Settings 7
Conclusions 8

2 Selecting Screening Scales: General Considerations   9

Evaluating Screening Scales 9
   Reliability and Validity 10
   Scale Validation 10
   Sensitivity and Specificity 10
What Type of Mistake Do You Prefer to Make? False Negatives vs.
   False Positives 10
Screening vs. Diagnosing 11
Conclusion 11

3 The Edinburgh Postnatal Depression Scale (EPDS)   12

Pros and Cons of the EPDS 12
Validation of the EPDS 13
Scale Cutoffs 14
   Low Cutoff: 9 to 11 14
   High Cutoff: 12 to 14+ 15

Variations of the EPDS 15
    The Edinburgh Postnatal Depression Scale-3 (EPDS-3) 16
    The Edinburgh Postnatal Depression Scale-2 (EPDS-2) 16
    EPDS-US 17
    EPDS-Partners and EPDS-Lifetime 17
Summary for Optimal Use of the EPDS 18

4 **The Patient Health Questionnaires**   19

Patient Health Questionnaire-9 (PHQ-9) 19
Patient Health Questionnaire-2 (PHQ-2) 20
Patient Health Questionnaire-4 (PHQ-4) 21

5 **Other Screening Tools**   23

The Postpartum Depression Screening Scale 23
The City Birth Trauma Scale 24
    Partner Version of the City Birth Trauma Scale 25
Patient Checklist for PTSD-DSM-5 (PCL-5) 26
Pittsburgh Sleep Quality Index (PSQI) 26
The Mood Disorder Questionnaire (MDQ) 27

6 **Assessing for Symptom Severity, Maternal Suicide Risk,
   and Possible Infant Harm**   28

Severity of the Current Episode 28
Suicide Risk 29
Possible Infant Harm 30

SECTION II
Complementary and Integrative Treatments   33

7 **An Integrative Approach to Treatment**   35

Mothers' Acceptance of Treatment 35
Complementary and Alternative Treatments for Depression 36
Do Non-Drug Treatments Work? 36

8 **Nutraceuticals I: Long-Chain Omega-3 Fatty Acids**   38

Omega-3s and Depression in Population Studies 39
Treatment with EPA and DHA 40
Effective Dosage of EPA 41
Why They Work: Stress, Inflammation, and EPA 42
DHA in the Perinatal Period 42
    DHA Lowers the Risk for Preterm Birth 43

Safety During Pregnancy and Lactation 43
  Pregnancy Studies 44
  Breastfeeding Studies 44
Sources of EPA and DHA 45
Summary 45

9 Nutraceuticals II: Vitamin D, Vitamin B-12, Curcumin, and St. John's Wort   47

Vitamin D 47
  Vitamin D and Postpartum Depression 48
Vitamin B-12 48
Curcumin 49
St. John's Wort 50
  Efficacy of St. John's Wort 50
  Mechanism for Efficacy 51
  Dosage 52
  Safety Concerns 52
  St. John's Wort and Breastfeeding 52
Summary 53

10 Exercise   55

Exercise as a Treatment for Depression 55
Exercise for Pregnant and Postpartum Women 56
Barriers to Exercise 57
Exercise Type 58
Exercise and Breastfeeding 59
Exercise Is Anti-Inflammatory 59

11 Bright Light Therapy   61

Light Therapy in Pregnant and Postpartum Women 61
Light Intensity, Duration, and Timing of Light Exposure 62
  Intensity 62
  Timing 63
  Dawn Simulation 63
Why Light Is Effective 63
Safety Issues 64

12 Emerging CAM Treatments   65

Acupuncture 65
Transcranial Direct Current Stimulation (tDCS) and Repetitive
  Transcranial Magnetic Stimulation (rTMS) 66
  Repetitive Transcranial Magnetic Stimulation 67
  Transcranial Direct Current Stimulation 67

SECTION III
Community Interventions   69

13 Social Support: The Foundation to Community Support   71

Support Lowers the Risk for Depression 72
What Is Effective Support? 73

14 Peer and Healthcare Provider Support   75

Identity of the Supporter: Peer or Professional? 75
  Peer Support 75
  Healthcare Provider Support 77
How Support Is Provided 78
  Telephone Support 78
  Digital Support 80

15 Home Visiting, Education, and Infant Massage   81

Home Visiting 81
Education 83
Infant Massage 84
Summary 86

SECTION IV
Psychotherapy   89

16 Cognitive-Behavioral Therapy   91

Mindfulness-Based Cognitive Therapy 93
  Self-Compassion 94
  Effectiveness Studies 95
The Anti-Inflammatory Effects of Cognitive Therapy 95

17 Interpersonal Psychotherapy   97

Clinical Trials and Perinatal Samples 98
Treatment for Partners 99
Long-Term Effects 99
Preventing Depression 99

18 Trauma-Informed Care and Trauma Treatment   101

Trauma-Informed Care 102
  SAMHSA's Six Key Principles of Trauma-Informed Care 103
Treatments for Trauma 104
  Cognitive-Processing Therapy (CPT) 104

Prolonged Exposure 105
Eye-Movement Desensitization and Reprocessing (EMDR) 105
Cognitive-Behavioral Therapy (CBT) 106
Medications 106
Complementary and Integrative Treatments for Trauma 107
Acupuncture 107
Mindfulness 108
Expressive Writing 108
Interventions Following Traumatic Childbirth 109
Debriefing 109
The Magical First Hour 110

SECTION V
Medications   113

19   Overview of Antidepressants   115

Psychosocial Considerations about Antidepressants 115
Selecting Which Medication to Use 116
Symptoms That Antidepressants Address 116
Mother's History 116
Depression Severity and Risk/Benefit Analysis in Treatment
Decisions 116
Typical Antidepressants 116
Tricyclics 117
Selective-Serotonin Reuptake Inhibitors (SSRIs) 117
Serotonin-Norepinephrine Reuptake Inhibitors 117
Norepinephrine–Dopamine Inhibitors 118
Monoamine Oxidase Inhibitors (MAOIs) 118
Phases of Depression Management with Medications 118
Acute Phase 118
Continuation Phase 119
Maintenance Phase 119
The Anti-Inflammatory Effects of Antidepressants 119

20   Antidepressants for Pregnant or Breastfeeding Women   121

In Utero Effects of Antidepressants 122
Antidepressants and Preterm Birth 122
First-Trimester Exposure 123
Third-Trimester Exposure and Discontinuation Syndrome 124
Childhood Effects of Pre- and Postnatal SSRI Exposure 124
Breastfeeding and Medications 126
Does Medication Cross into Breastmilk? 127
The Bottom Line 127

21 Atypical Antidepressants: Ketamine and Brexanolone 129

GABA and Glutamate 129
Ketamine 130
   Esketamine 130
   Ketamine Use in Postpartum Women 131
Brexanolone 132
   Efficacy 133
   Limitations of Brexanolone 134
   Zuranolone 134

22 Putting It All Together 135

References 137
Index 163

Foreword

It is a privilege to contribute this Foreword to Dr. Kendall-Tackett's book on screening, assessment, and treatment for depression in new mothers. This book is a critical step forward in providing evidence-based research to inform clinical assessment and practice. Novel in many of its ideas and rich in studies with culturally diverse populations, it is a book that anyone who studies or treats new moms with depression will find informative and an essential read.

I began treating moms with maternal depression back in 1987, before I had my first baby. Although I'd been counseling other women about the importance of self-care and other skills for coping with becoming a mom, I hadn't been practicing them myself. I learned firsthand how new moms struggle to adjust to this life-altering change and what a profound effect it has on us. It was a defining moment for me, resulting in my choosing maternal/perinatal mental health and women's reproductive health psychology as the focus of my clinical practice.

I attended my first Postpartum Support International (PSI) conference in 1988 and became part of the initial group of advocates and practitioners to promote awareness and education about maternal depression, which has a major impact on the health and well-being of both moms and babies. In 1994, I co-authored my first book with Dr. Anne Dunnewold on what we then called postpartum depression, *Postpartum Survival Guide*. Since then, I have co-authored 2 more books on perinatal mental/emotional health and treated hundreds of women and their families for what we also call "the most frequent complication of childbirth."

Back then, we worked tirelessly to educate both the lay public and professional health community that depression in new moms existed and that if it went un- or under-treated, moms, babies, and families would suffer. There was much resistance to the idea that motherhood might not lead to bliss and could result in depression. It took decades to get depression in new moms recognized as a "real" health condition and for organizations including the American Academy of Pediatrics and the American College of Obstetrics and Gynecology to create guidelines for screening and referral of perinatal women. Still, there is room for improvement, and Dr. Kendall-Tackett's book offers an evidence-based toolkit for screening, assessment, and treatment suggestions.

Coming from a developmental psychology background, Dr. Kendall-Tackett understood how much a new mom's relationship with her baby impacted her baby's development and was always curious about how differences in a mother's psychological health status affected her infant. After becoming a mom herself, she became interested in the topic and wrote the first edition of this book. After her second baby, she became a volunteer for La Leche League, the premiere organization that supports breastfeeding moms.

In this role, she met thousands of new mothers and learned about the qualitative experience of the postpartum period. Over time, she became an expert in the study of breast-feeding and has published extensively on this topic, particularly on its interactions with maternal mental health.

While I was practicing clinical assessment and treatment of depression in new moms, Kathy was doing research and writing articles on maternal mental health. She was also talked to hundreds of new moms about the impact of birth trauma on breastfeeding and the effects of a mother's early childhood abuse/trauma on her birth and postpartum adjustment. Although she will tell you that she's not clinically trained, her ability to listen to moms and take what she's learned and turn it into quantitative research is noteworthy.

Dr. Kendall-Tackett's newest book is a compilation of 30+ years of formal and informal study of new moms and her comprehensive review of current research on screening, assessment, and treatment of depression in new moms. Her ideas about how inflammatory processes contribute to maternal mental health changes are thought-provoking. She provides evidence-based studies that support an integrated, multi-modal approach to care that takes cultural considerations and issues of community accessibility to health resources into account. She talks about what's working, what's not, and how we can do better. It is a valuable addition to the library of any clinician or researcher who is interested in or works in the field of maternal mental health.

I hope that you will study and learn from this book, as I have. It is with much respect and gratitude that I offer this foreword to Dr. Kathleen A. Kendall-Tackett for her commitment to the field of maternal mental health and supporting moms and babies to create healthier families and communities.

Dr. Diane Sanford, Psychologist, Author, and Educator Specializing in
Women's Reproductive Mental Health
St. Louis, Missouri

Preface

Over the years, I have seen what individuals and small organizations can do when they decide to help depressed new mothers. Communities can implement effective interventions and use resources that are already available. In *Depression in New Mothers, Volume I*, I described risk factors for depression and its consequences, and the conditions that often co-occur, such as anxiety and PTSD. Volume II will help you assess and either treat depression or make a referral for treatment.

Even if you are not a mental health provider, there is much you can do. I frequently speak at hospitals and educate nurses, lactation consultants, and childbirth educators. After I had been with them, I learned that they started programs where new mothers get together (social support) to walk outside with their babies (exercise, bright light, and Vitamin D). They also take omega-3s. With these simple interventions, depression rates at these various hospitals plummeted. That is just one example of how these studies can be applied. These programs used resources already available and were able to influence mothers' mental health in some dramatic ways.

Unfortunately, I have also seen bad examples of what happens out in the field, where practitioners engage in "magical thinking" about depression. They think that by simply administering the "Edinberg" (referring to the Edinburgh Postnatal Depression Scale[1]), they have "fixed" depression. When I ask, "What happens when a mother screens positive?" I get blank stares. In the meantime, mothers who are screened may believe that help is on the way. Instead, all they hear is silence. They conclude that no one cares. Screening is useless without follow-up. And mothers should be assessed until they no longer have symptoms (Yeaton-Massey & Herrero, 2019).

The Next Steps: What Happens after Screening?

According to the US Preventive Services Task Force, screening for depression should take place in a context where there are adequate systems in place to ensure accurate diagnosis, effective treatment, and appropriate follow-up (O'Connor et al., 2016). Yeaton-Massey and Herrero (2019) concur and recommend education, support, and timely referral to resources. In practical terms, this means figuring out what to do if a mother screens positive.

Think for a moment. If you had a program for depression in new mothers, what would it look like? Who else would be involved? What resources can you leverage? I encourage you to describe your dream program. Based on what is available, can you assemble the resources you need? You may need to tweak the final version of your vision, but writing it out will help you think it through. Consider the following:

- What scale will you use to assess depression, and what cutoff will signal that intervention is necessary?
- What communities do you work with? What types of treatments are most acceptable within your community? This is especially important to think about when your population includes mothers of different ethnicities and nationalities.
- Will you treat mothers who screen positive, or will you refer them to other programs?
- What options are available to mothers right away?
- Do mothers need other types of help, such as food and housing assistance, lactation support, domestic violence services, or trauma treatment programs? What groups can help with those needs?

No matter the treatment course, follow-up and repeated assessment are critical. Too often, I have met mothers who were sent home with a prescription and no follow-up. The medication was not effective (as is true for 30% to 40% of patients who take them), yet the practitioner believed that they had "treated" depression. They had not. Follow-up with further assessment must be part of the plan.

Traditional vs. Innovative Treatments for Depression in New Mothers

The field has changed so much in the past 30 years. Back in the 1990s, medications were the only treatment option, with psychotherapy sometimes offered as an adjunct. This treatment model was based on the experiences of White middle-class mothers who saw psychiatrists.

Fortunately, we now have a lot more choice. However, many practitioners are not aware of all the innovative treatments available and seem stuck in the 1990s. For example, this recent article (Stewart & Vigod, 2019) suggests that alternative treatments, such as exercise, self-care, and social support, only work for mild depression. For moderate or severe depression, *medications are the only thing that work*. If depression does not remit, you can add electroconvulsive therapy (ECT). O'Hara and Engeldinger (2018) added psychotherapy as a possible option.

The most recent *Clinical Practice Guidelines* from the American College of Obstetricians and Gynecologists offers specific treatment recommendations for depression, anxiety, bipolar disorder, and psychosis, "with a focus on psychopharmacology" (American College of Obstetricians and Gynecologists, 2023). Another article either dismissed or did not mention non-pharmacologic treatments for depression (Kimmel et al., 2018). They concluded that medications are the only real option:

> Although there have not been any randomized controlled trials of psychotherapy vs pharmacotherapy for perinatal depression, epidemiologic data suggest that for moderate to severe symptoms, *psychotherapy alone may not be sufficient, and augmentation with pharmacotherapy ought to be considered.*
>
> (p. 431, emphasis added)

As I will demonstrate, this statement is simply not true. Time after time, psychotherapy has proven to be as effective as medications in even severe depression. I present the evidence on the efficacy of psychotherapy in Chapters 16–18. And there are many other options. Treatment for depression has radically changed over the past 30 years.

I encourage you to read these pages with an open mind. I hope these chapters will give you many great ideas that will benefit mothers in your community. Treatment is, perhaps, where the field has made its greatest strides. Volume II presents the evidence that will allow you to customize your treatment approach. The more options you have, the more effective you will be.

Moving Ahead

This is an exciting time to be in the postpartum depression field. The evidence base is large, but the need is even greater. My aim is to help you evaluate assessment tools and treatment options and select the ones that will work best for the mothers you serve. Depression in new mothers is a global problem, and studies on treatment options come from around the world. There is literally something for everyone.

With this information, *you* can make a difference in the lives of young families, alone or in collaboration with others. So much can be done at the community level. My aim is to equip you to do just that.

Kathleen A. Kendall-Tackett, PhD, IBCLC, FAPA
Amarillo, Texas, August 20, 2023

Note

1 This is a peeve of mine. The EPDS is named for Edinburgh (Ed-in-burr-ah), the Scottish city where it was created. No Scot calls it "Edinberg." However, we do have an Edinberg near where I live in Texas.

Section I

Screening for Depression and CoMorbid Conditions

1 Screening

Rationale and Barriers

Screening for depression is the vital first step; you cannot treat depression if you do not know that it exists. Unfortunately, if practitioners do not screen, they will not learn that some of their new mothers are depressed, and will not be able to help. This chapter describes why screening is helpful and why those who want to screen often encounter barriers.

KEY FINDINGS

- Health organizations recommend screening mothers for depression, but most new mothers are never screened.
- Barriers include time constraints, not having clearly identified steps when there is a positive screen, fear of "opening Pandora's box," and believing that they can identify depression without a validated scale.

Why Screening Is Helpful

The US Agency for Healthcare Research and Quality (ARHQ) noted that screening increases the likelihood that postpartum depression can be prevented or treated (Myers et al., 2013). ARHQ outlined the components necessary for a screening strategy. The key components are:

1. Which screening scale to use
2. When to screen
3. Who should screen
4. How to use the results of the screening test

ARHQ noted that while most major health organizations concede that screening is important, their recommendations vary. For example, the American College of Obstetricians and Gynecologists Committee on Obstetric Practice (2023) notes that "routine screening by physicians is important for ensuring appropriate follow-up and treatment." The UK National Institute for Health and Clinical Excellence (NICE) has a more effective policy in that it specifically recommends who should screen (the primary provider), when it should happen (at the first contact, at 4 to 6 weeks or 3 to 4 months), which professionals should do it (all), and what to ask. These guidelines recommend the Edinburgh Postnatal Depression Scale, the Patient Health Questionnaire-9, and the Hospital Anxiety and Depression Scale (HADS).

DOI: 10.4324/9781003405092-2

Barriers to Screening

Despite recommendations, healthcare providers are far more likely to screen for gestational diabetes, which occurs in 2.4% of mothers, and pregnancy-associated hypertension, which occurs in 5.5% of pregnancies (McGarry et al., 2009), than they are for depression. Conservative estimates of depression during pregnancy are 15% to 25% (Grigoriadis et al., 2018; Staneva et al., 2015). In the United States, this clinical torpor is of particular concern for African American mothers, where depression is often missed and it increases the risk for preterm birth (Nutor et al., 2018).

Why would healthcare providers be reluctant to screen? The "Pandora's box" dilemma is one barrier. Lack of resources is another. In Canada, their current health recommendations are against universal screening because potential false positives could "overly burden" their primary care providers (Lang et al., 2022). Surprisingly, they did not think that screening was superior to usual care. Yet 23% of their mothers have either postpartum depression or anxiety, according to Statistics Canada (2019). These numbers suggest that "usual care" is not effective.

Screening can also be an equity issue. In US samples, ethnic minority women are often not screened for depression. When they are included, they often have much higher rates of depression, anxiety, and PTSD. For example, the Listening to Mothers in California study included 2,539 women based on a representative sample of birth certificate files (Declercq et al., 2021). They used the Patient Health Questionnaire-4 (PHQ-4) and asked whether mothers were receiving counseling or taking medication for depression or anxiety. In their sample, non-Latina Black women had higher postpartum depressive symptoms and lower use of medication or counseling compared to non-Latina White women. Women who were screened were 6 times more likely to receive counseling. The authors concluded that their findings argue for universal screening to reduce inequities and help address underuse of counseling, especially for women of color.

Many studies on screening take place in either pediatric or obstetric settings. In some ways, healthcare providers are in a perfect place to screen for depression; mothers have multiple contacts with them. However, barriers exist in healthcare settings too.

One barrier is providers' belief that they are good at identifying depression without using a validated scale. Studies show that most are not, and their observations are often highly inaccurate (Hilt, 2015). Validated scales are more accurate, and according to US national guidelines, they need to be administered regularly throughout the first year (Siu & US Preventive Services Task Force (USPSTF), 2016).

Screening scales can also help mothers who are unwilling to tell healthcare providers that they are depressed. For example, 66% of women with depressive symptoms in the Utah PRAMS[1] study did not seek help (McGarry et al., 2009). A review of 40 studies found the same thing. In addition, family members and health professionals often reinforced mothers' lack of help-seeking by minimizing their symptoms or saying that they were normal (Dennis & Chung-Lee, 2006). Mothers listened and hoped that depression would get better on its own. Mothers also feared that authorities would take their babies away. This is a rare but realistic concern. It has even happened in my community. This fear is a significant barrier to determining whether a new mother is depressed. Finally, many mothers are ashamed of being depressed (Sword et al., 2008).

A review of 23 studies ($N = 5,398$) considered whether screening pregnant and postpartum women in primary care was helpful or harmful (O'Connor et al., 2016). In postpartum women, screening reduced overall prevalence of depression and increased the likelihood of treatment or remission. The authors expressed some concerns that women with previous depressions were excluded from studies, noting that they would also benefit from screening. Screening also allowed clinicians to ask mothers about suicidal ideations and refer them for treatment. The evidence suggests that screening pregnant and postpartum women reduces depressive symptoms and prevalence within a given population, especially if screening is followed by treatment and clinical care.

Screening in Pediatric Settings

For many mothers in the United States, pediatricians are the most logical people to screen for postpartum depression. A pediatrician will see mothers up to 7 times in the first year for well-baby visits alone (Currie & Rademacher, 2004; Freeman et al., 2005; Heneghan et al., 2007). Depressed mothers may avoid getting care for themselves but will get care for their babies. The barrier is that many pediatricians are not trained in adult medicine and do not feel qualified to handle the mothers' mental health. "Pandora's box" is another reason that they do not screen. A pediatrician with a busy practice may feel that they do not have time to "deal" with a depressed mother. A few years ago, I did a training for pediatric residents on depression at our local medical school. The chief pediatric resident said, "I don't know what this has to do with pediatrics." Unfortunately, many clinicians I know have encountered have the same attitude. When pediatricians understand that mothers' mental health directly influences infants, they are more likely to participate in screening and referral.

The good news is that the American Academy of Pediatrics (AAP) has officially acknowledged maternal mental health as important for pediatricians and affirmed that they should screen (Earls & The Committee on Psychosocial Aspects of Child and Family Health, 2010; Rafferty et al., 2019). Ideally, screening will be followed by referrals to someone who can help.

> Perinatal depression is a pertinent issue for the primary care clinician because of the significant risks to the health and well-being of the infant and the family. Pediatric primary care practices . . . can build a system to implement postpartum depression screening, to connect affected families to supportive community resources, and to refer parents for additional treatment when indicated.
>
> (Rafferty et al., 2019, p. 11)

The AAP notes that depression increases the risk of breastfeeding cessation, family dysfunction, and even child maltreatment. Screening and referral to resources in the community are key to supporting healthy attachment and parent–child relationships (Rafferty et al., 2019).

In Alberta, Canada, mothers were screened at immunization clinics, with data collected during 2012 ($N = 51,537$) and 2016 ($N = 55,787$) using the Edinburgh Postnatal Depression Scale (McPhail et al., 2021). The percentage of mothers screened decreased between 2012 (80%) and 2016 (70%). Mothers were less likely to be screened if they were older than 29. For some strange reason, mothers 35 and older were the least likely to be screened. In contrast to previous studies, lower-income mothers were *more* likely to be screened. That focus is appropriate, but screening should be for all mothers, including older ones.

A Turkish study screened at well-child visits and found that 34% of mothers were in the clinical range on the EPDS at 1 month postpartum (Orhon et al., 2007).

Mothers with depressive symptoms had more negative perceptions of their infants and reported more fussing, crying, sleep, and temperament problems. When mothers' depression was treated, their sleep and perception of their infants improved. Depressed mothers were more likely to report insufficient milk during the first 2 months, but breastfeeding initiation was 100%, with high continuation rates even among the depressed mothers.

Barriers to Screening

Although screening is effective, relatively few pediatricians do it. The American Academy of Pediatrics' guidelines note that the percentage of pediatricians screening for postpartum depression is slowly increasing, from 13% to 47% (Rafferty et al., 2019). Head and colleagues (2008) acknowledged that pediatricians were in an ideal position to detect maternal depression, but few of the 1,600 AAP members they surveyed were trained to do it. Residents had the highest percentage of training, but it was only 20%. Older pediatricians had the least amount of trainings and the lowest level of interest in mothers' mental health. Even with residency reforms, 81% of current residents had no training in adult mental health issues.

Heneghan and colleagues (2007) asked 662 pediatricians how they identified and managed maternal depression. Seventy-seven percent had identified at least one depressed mother, and 82% of those had referred the mother to services. (They did not say what happened to the 18% of mothers not referred to services.) Pediatricians were more likely to identify depression if:

1. Their practice provides child mental health services.
2. They thought that maternal mental health influenced child health.
3. They believed it was their job to identify and manage maternal depression.

A focus group of 27 new mothers with a history of depression described the barriers to care they encountered in pediatric settings (Byatt et al., 2013). Mothers did not want pediatricians to judge them or think they would kill their babies. Mothers also reported that providers were not knowledgeable and that they minimized mothers' concerns. However, when pediatricians listened empathically and offered tangible referrals and resources, mothers felt empowered.

MedEdPPD offers a free Care Pathways document designed for physicians and other primary care healthcare providers who want to learn who to screen and refer mothers for treatment, complete with treatment algorithms (www.MedEdPPD.com) (Wisner et al., 2008). Pediatricians are not the prime people who should treat depression, but they can be the gateway to care and should know where to send mothers for help in their communities. They might even have their staff help mothers schedule appointments, as mothers sometimes have difficulty navigating this system and reaching out for help. In a study of 2,199 pregnant women, 19% had a cutoff >9 (mild depression), and 5% had an EPDS >14 (severe depression), using the Edinburgh Postnatal Depression Scale (EPDS). Yet only 1 woman pursued follow-up referrals. At 6 weeks, 28 women screened positive for depression, and only 5 followed up with behavioral healthcare referrals (McClellan et al., 2012). If depressed women do not seek care after being screened, a different approach may be needed, including discussing self-care and other non-medical, non-pharmacologic treatments.

Screening in Obstetric Settings

Obstetricians are another prime group to screen and treat new mothers. The mothers are their patients. They come in for a 6-week check (earlier if they had cesareans). And yet obstetricians are not likely to do it.

The current guidelines from the American College of Obstetricians and Gynecologists (2015) and the US Preventive Services Task Force (Siu & US Preventive Services Task Force (USPSTF), 2016) recommend that all perinatal women be screened at least once during the perinatal period for depression and anxiety using a standardized instrument. Unfortunately, this guideline to screen "at least once" may be too limited to accurately detect depression and anxiety in the perinatal period, but most are not doing even that. O'Hara and Engeldinger (2018) noted the following:

> The sad reality is that large numbers of women suffer from mental health disorders during their childbearing years. The obstetrician-gynecologist is the only primary care provider for many women and has great responsibility to address the mental health of patients along with their physical health during and after pregnancy.
>
> (p. 613)

A study of 19 obstetricians and 3 midwives found that most respondents acknowledged that screening was important but few consistently did it (Kim et al., 2009). Ninety-five percent of the providers overestimated their rates of screening, and 67% thought they had achieved universal screening. However, the results showed something far different. If providers did not directly screen (i.e., had their staff do it), only 37% did it. If they did it themselves, 59% actively screened. One barrier was no office prompt to remind them to screen. Others were concerned about giving the PPD screen to everyone ("not everyone needs this"), that there was no time to do it, or that they lacked expertise to handle mental health issues. Higher screening rates depended on more active provider commitment.

An interesting follow-up study found that the ACOG screening guidelines did not increase the percentage of depressed women identified (Leboffe et al., 2023). The before-and-after-guidelines percentages were 15% and 17%, respectively, controlling for age, year, delivery complications, and geographic region. The samples were large: $N = 414,890$ women pre-guideline, and $N = 77,662$ post-guideline. ACOG concluded that prior to 2015, there was no reason to recommend universal screening for PPD. (This recommendation is astonishing in that there is more than 30 years' worth of studies documenting incidence and harmful effects of postpartum depression.) The relatively low percentages of women identified are also interesting and could be related to how they were identified. Women were classified as depressed if they had an ICD diagnosis for postpartum or other depression or a prescription for antidepressants in the first 12 months postpartum. Both measures would miss many depressed women. Very few women are even screened, much less diagnosed. In addition, many depressed women never get a prescription. The authors of the ACOG guidelines noted that general practitioners, pediatricians, and psychiatrists are not influenced by the ACOG screening guidelines. The authors suggested education and addressing barriers to make screening more effective.

Interestingly, obstetricians were significantly more confident than pediatricians that they could identify depression without a scale. In a survey and chart-review study, all 47 survey respondents agreed that it was their responsibility to screen for depression, and 94% were confident that they could diagnose it. Far fewer were actually doing it.

Obstetric providers charted the Edinburgh Postnatal Depression Scales (EPDS) score in 39% of the visits and counseled their patients in 35% of the visits (Delatte et al., 2009). There was a significant difference in referral rates, depending on the provider. Residents had the lowest rates (17%). This is discouraging since we might assume that younger physicians would be more likely to refer. Forty-two percent of attendings referred, compared to 67% of certified nurse midwives and 94% of nurse practitioners. This study was designed to evaluate the effectiveness of a policy of universal screening at a local medical center. The researchers noted that their results highlight the gap between what providers know should be done and what was actually done at postpartum visits.

Conclusions

Although professional organizations indicate that screening is important, it is far from universal. For both pediatricians and obstetricians, barriers include lack of training about depression in general and what to do with a positive result, short office visits and tight scheduling, and the possibility of opening "Pandora's box," Believing that mothers will "fall apart" when they reveal that they are depressed. Many obstetricians and pediatricians believe that this is not within their purview to screen and refer for depression, so it is not likely to happen. A lesson learned from research on domestic violence is that screening is more likely to occur when practitioners are educated about it and know what to do when a patient screens positive, when there are "prompts" to do it (such as appearing in electronic medical records), and when administrators follow up to make sure that it was done. Without those constraints, screening is less likely to happen.

The good news is that organizations outside of the medical world have begun screening for depression. It is easy for them to do it since most of the scales are available for free online. In addition, screening and referring mothers to community resources is well within the scope of practice of many non-medical, non–mental health practitioners.

Clinical Takeaways

- Screening is a necessary first step to treatment. Mothers cannot be treated if practitioners do not know they are depressed.
- Simply "mandating" screening is unlikely to increase compliance. Providers need to understand why it is relevant to their clinical practice and there should be institutional support to ensure compliance.
- Electronic prompts for providers can increase screening in health settings. But there also needs to be a clear plan for what happens when mothers screen positive. Providers are more likely to screen if they know what to do next.

Note

1 PRAMS = Pregnancy Risk Assessment Monitoring Study.

2 Selecting Screening Scales
General Considerations

Selecting a screening scale is the first step in any intervention for depression and co-occurring conditions. There are many screening scales that are widely available, and they are all helpful in identifying depression, anxiety, and PTSD. This chapter will help you evaluate the available measures and select the one most appropriate for your population.

KEY FINDINGS

- No scale is perfect, but metrics such as reliability and validity can help you judge whether it is appropriate for you to use.
- A scale's sensitivity and specificity are two constructs directly related to your screening goals. *Sensitivity* is a scale's ability to detect symptoms. *Specificity* refers to its ability to only identify mothers with a specific condition, such as major depression, but not milder symptoms. If you want to identify mothers with mild or moderate symptoms, then high sensitivity is important. If you only want mothers with major depression, higher specificity is important.

I recommend also screening for co-occurring anxiety and PTSD, and possibly bipolar disorder. Anxiety is particularly prominent. A Croatian study found that pregnancy was a high-risk time for anxiety, with or without comorbid depression (Rados et al., 2018). In their sample of 272 new mothers, 35% had anxiety during pregnancy, 17% had anxiety immediately postpartum, and 21% had anxiety at 6 weeks. Seventy-five percent of mothers with anxiety were also depressed. However, if mothers were only screened for depression, the 25% who had anxiety only would not have been identified.

Evaluating Screening Scales

The American Academy of Pediatrics recommends the Edinburgh Postnatal Depression Scale (EPDS), the Patient Health Questionnaire-2 (PHQ-2), the Patient Health Questionnaire-9 (PHQ-9), and the Postpartum Depression Screening Scale (PDSS) (Earls & The Committee on Psychosocial Aspects of Child and Family Health, 2010; Rafferty et al., 2019). Similarly, the US Preventive Services Task Force recommends the Edinburgh Postnatal Depression Scale and the Patient Health Questionnaires (all versions) (Siu & US

DOI: 10.4324/9781003405092-3

Preventive Services Task Force (USPSTF), 2016). A recent review in the American Family Physician noted that:

> Women should be screened for depression at least once during the perinatal period using the PHQ-2, PHQ-9, or Edinburgh Postnatal Depression Scale.
>
> (Maurer et al., 2018, p. 508)

I will describe these scales in subsequent chapters, but before I do, I want to briefly describe criteria researchers use to judge the merits of a particular scale. These are the factors that researchers describe when discussing a scale in the literature.

Reliability and Validity

Reliability and validity of a scale are critical metrics to determine whether a scale is a viable choice. Does it measure what it says it does (construct validity)? Are the results consistent when administered to the same person more than once (test-retest reliability)? Does it have internal consistency (Cronbach's alpha)? These metrics are frequently cited in validation studies.

Scale Validation

How was the scale was developed? When the authors developed the scale, whom did they test it on? Is that group relevant to new mothers? For example, if the scale was validated on White men, it might not be appropriate for women, particularly ethnic minority women. It might still be effective, but there would be concern until it was also validated on a sample of perinatal women.

Sensitivity and Specificity

Studies also report a scale's specificity and sensitivity. *Sensitivity* means it detects most possible cases. *Specificity* means that it only identifies people with the condition in question and not people with other conditions. High specificity means it will not identify a mother as depressed when she is not. These scales will identify mothers with severe depression but miss mothers with mild or moderate symptoms. If you want to identify everyone that is at risk, including those with mild or moderate symptoms, high sensitivity is more important (Myers et al., 2013).

What Type of Mistake Do You Prefer to Make? False Negatives vs. False Positives

Postpartum depression studies debate whether screening should encompass mild to moderate depression (and some possible false positives) or only identify mothers with major depression (and possibly some false negatives). This is the difference of Type 1 vs. Type 2 errors. A Type 1 error may falsely identify a mother as depressed when if she is not but would identify women with mild or moderate symptoms. In contrast, with a Type 2 error, you miss some cases of depression but only identify mothers with severe symptoms.

In the context of screening for depression in new mothers, Type 1 vs. 2 errors are usually focused on cutoff scores that should be used on the Edinburgh Postnatal Depression Scale (EPDS). What seems like a methodological quibble (should you use a low vs. high cutoff?) has real-world consequences. A more stringent definition (higher cutoff) means not identifying mothers with mild or moderate symptoms (lower cutoff). Given your community and the constraints of your resources, which is preferable? Identifying some mothers as depressed when they are not or missing mothers with mild or moderate symptoms?

With false positives, you may overestimate the prevalence of a condition, which may lead to allocating more resources than you need. Conversely, Dennis et al. (2004a) argue that false negatives are far more costly, and therefore, they recommend using a lower cutoff. These studies are described in more detail in Chapter 3.

Screening vs. Diagnosing

Once a person has screened positive, an in-depth assessment tool should be used to make a diagnosis. Unfortunately, that rarely happens. In many contexts, screening scales are the sole assessment. They can function that way, but I need to acknowledge that they are not supposed to. This is particularly true with the most widely used assessment tool: the Edinburgh Postnatal Depression Scale.

Screening vs. diagnosis also influences the results of incidence studies. Screening scales cast a wide net over possible mothers who might be depressed, so incidence rates appear higher than they do when a diagnostic tool, such as the Center for Epidemiologic Studies-Depression (CES-D), which is far more stringent, is used.

In subsequent chapters, I describe commonly used scales in detail. Because of copyright concerns, I have not been able to include versions of these scales in this book, but most are freely available online; a simple Google search will yield the scale and its scoring instructions.

Conclusion

Mothers often do not reveal that they are depressed unless specifically asked. They may not even realize that they are depressed, but they often know that *something* is wrong. You can screen for depression by using one of the standardized screening measures. Screening can also help you determine whether a mother is suicidal, needs to be hospitalized, or needs a referral for other assistance.

Once depression has been identified, mothers need to be treated. There is a wide range of treatments available for depressed new mothers. These are described in detail in Sections II to V.

Clinical Takeaways

- No scale is perfect, but many are very good. The population you serve, the reading level, the time it takes to complete, and the ease of access are all relevant in choosing an assessment tool. You may decide to use more than one.
- Think through the goals of screening to help you determine whether a broad or narrow screen is more appropriate. If you only want to identify mothers with major depression, a more stringent measure is appropriate. If you want to identify all depression, a broader screen is appropriate.
- For programs in community settings, a broader screen is generally appropriate. If, however, resources are scarce, a more stringent measure would be a better choice.

3   The Edinburgh Postnatal Depression Scale (EPDS)

The Edinburgh Postnatal Depression Scale (EPDS) is the most widely used screening tool for postpartum depression in the world. The EPDS is a 10-item self-report questionnaire that can be completed in 5 minutes (Cox et al., 1987). The original intent was that primary healthcare providers would administer it (Cox, 2019), but it is used in every setting and context imaginable and often does not include a healthcare provider at all. With the scale, women are asked to report how they have felt *in the past week*, and each item is scored from 0 to 3. The authors have granted use of their questionnaire without charge or permission if the source of the scale is listed and the copyright is respected. Interestingly, shortened versions of the EPDS are often more sensitive and focus particularly on anxiety symptoms within the scale (Walker et al., 2015). The EPDS has been validated with samples of adult women around the world and has been translated into many languages.

KEY FINDINGS

- The EPDS is used worldwide. It is appropriate for both research and practice.
- It has been validated in many studies, with a range of mothers.
- Lower cutoffs on the EPDS are for broad screening. Higher cutoffs will only identify mothers with severe depression.
- Limitations of the EPDS include language and scoring issues. Some researchers have also noted difficulty translating the EPDS because it uses expressions that are particular to colloquial British English, so literal translation may not make sense for mothers outside the UK or the Commonwealth. A recent iteration of the EPDS (EPDS-US) addressed these language issues but it has not yet been validated.
- The EPDS-3 has better reliability and validity than the full version.

Pros and Cons of the EPDS

The EPDS offers several advantages. It is easy to complete and score. Mothers can answer all the questions in a few minutes, and it is specifically for new mothers. Indeed, the EPDS was developed to address the limitations of more generic depression measures. From a research perspective, it is easy to justify its use in that most studies use it, which makes it easier to compare results.

Lappin (2001) notes that the EPDS was designed to be used in the early postpartum period, has been validated for that use, and should not be used for screening for depression in pregnancy or to diagnose depression beyond the postpartum period. In the real world, it is often used for both. Lappin (2001) also cautions against interpreting one- to

DOI: 10.4324/9781003405092-4

two-point differences to mean increased severity. Lappin noted that this instrument is best at predicting depression with a cutoff of 12.

Another unknown is whether the EPDS is useful for minority populations in the United States. Heck (2018) reviewed 58 articles that examined validation of the EPDS and PHQ-9. Both measures have good internal consistency, but she found that it missed depression in minority populations, such as American Indians and Alaska Natives. She believes that both the EPDS and PHQ might be culturally biased toward educated White women.

The EPDS contains several items with reverse scoring, making it easy to mis-score items. Matthey et al. (2013) collected 496 EPDSs from client files and examined them for scoring errors from 6 practices in Australia. They also surveyed 22 clinicians and asked them to estimate the rate of errors. Clinicians made many more mistakes than they realized. Matthey et al. found that 17% of the forms had at least one error, where clinicians tallied the score incorrectly. Most were off by only one point, which generally did not make a difference. However, there was some concern because being off by one point could make the difference between a positive and negative screen for depression. The authors noted that the EPDS is not easy to manually score despite claims that it is.

Validation of the EPDS

Validation is the process by which researchers determine whether a scale measures what it purports to measure. In this process, the new measure is compared to established ones that do measure the construct (in this case, depression). If a new scale identifies roughly the same percentage of people as depressed, researchers believe that it is a valid measure of depression. However, when looking at validation studies, it is important to keep in mind that screening scales do not have the same goals as diagnostic instruments. Screening scales are trying to pick up on depressive symptoms and are not designed to diagnose major depressive disorder. Ones that are more focused on only major depression will have a smaller prevalence rate. That does not mean that the screening scale is invalid; it simply has a different function. However, a more stringent cutoff should be consistent with diagnostic scales for major depression since a higher cutoff usually means more severe symptoms. Cox (2019) noted that the EPDS cannot provide a differential diagnosis for either anxiety or PTSD (although shorter versions of the EDPS are good screening tools for anxiety; these are described in subsequent sections).

The EPDS has been validated by comparing it to measures such as the Center for Epidemiologic Studies-Depression Scale (CES-D), a 20-item diagnostic scale for depression (Logsdon et al., 2009). When used in the first 6 weeks, the EPDS has equivalent performance to the Hamilton Depression Rating Scale-17 and 21, and the Beck Depression Inventory when using optimal cutoffs (Myers et al., 2013).

Previous studies have noted that the EPDS measures not only depression but also other disorders, such as anxiety. One way to determine if there are other conditions that the EPDS measures is to run confirmatory factor analyses on the various models presented in these previous studies. King (2012) used the EPDS as a screening tool for 169 low-income African American women, a group typically underrepresented in postpartum depression studies. She found high rates of depression with her sample. When the cutoff was >10, 30% screened positive for depression, and 19% did when the cutoff was >13. With confirmatory factor analysis, she found that the three-factor model with depression, anxiety, and anhedonia was the best fit for her sample. These findings suggest that anxiety and anhedonia are distinct from depression and are relevant for this sample.

A review of 16 studies with mothers in low- to middle-income countries (LMIC) aggregated findings from 12 countries in 14 languages (Shrestha et al., 2016). The sample included 1,281 mothers. They found that most local-language versions were less precise than the original English version. Of the studies, only one had a culturally sensitive translation. The authors noted deficiencies in translation, cultural adaptation, and validation processes. But most studies simply translated the original language, and the questions might not have been understood because the diagnostic protocol had not been culturally adapted such that a literal translation of these scales might cause mothers with little education to not understand, whereas mothers with higher education levels could when local expressions were used in the translations. Two studies used culturally appropriate wording and almost doubled their sensitivity. In addition, the scales are often validated using mothers recruited from prenatal clinics, who tend to be more educated. Those translations may not be effective with mothers with low literacy. The authors recommended that translations explicitly consider local terminology for psychological distress and mental health disorders. They also recommended that researchers consider literacy level and that cutoff scores be validated for each culture, along with culturally validated standard diagnostic protocol. An inaccurate measure may mean that mothers with depression do not get identified, or mothers who are not depressed may be labeled as having it, creating an unnecessary burden on often-overtaxed healthcare systems.

I find the "translation" issues to be a concern even when comparing American vs. British English. For example, some questions on the EPDS are oddly worded for American mothers (e.g., "[T]hings are getting on top of me lately"). I understand why making a word-for-word translation, without considering how mothers in a culture describe themselves as overwhelmed, would not accurately assess how they were feeling. Cox (2019), as author of the scale, also noted that nuances of language and meaning of metaphors can change over time. Interestingly, he also pointed out that the "[T]hings have been getting on top of me" item was challenging for mothers who do not speak British English. The recent U.S version of the EPDS may address some of these concerns (Moyer et al., 2023).

Scale Cutoffs

The cutoff used on the EPDS can vary depending on its intended purpose: broad screening or to identify only women with more serious depressions. The standard cutoff is 12 for depression (Cox, 2019), but higher and lower cutoffs have been used. The justification for different cutoffs depends on the user's goal. Lower cutoffs may include women who are not depressed, while higher cutoffs identify women with severe depression but miss others with less severe symptoms.

Low Cutoff: 9 to 11

Dennis (2004a, 2004b) found that using 9 as a cutoff increased the sensitivity of the scale, which makes it more appropriate for community screening (Dennis, 2004a). In contrast, a higher cutoff has more specificity but may miss some depressed women. In her study of 594 women, a cutoff of 12/13 at week 1 missed depression in 43% of mothers at 4 weeks, and 53% of mothers at 8 weeks.

A study validated the Danish version of the EPDS against the DSM-5 and the ICD-10 diagnostic criteria for postpartum depression (Smith-Nielsen et al., 2018). Their sample included 324 women at 2 and 10 months. They used the Structured Clinical

Interview-Depression. Eleven was the optimal cutoff for both DSM-5 and ICD-10 criteria. They noted that this cutoff was not validated for a prenatal sample and suggested that it should be before it is used.

Smith-Nielsen (2018) identified three factors in the EPDS—depression (items 1, 2, 8, 9), anxiety (items 3, 4, and 5), and self-harm/suicide (item 10)—but noted that the variation in different studies may reflect differences in how mothers reflect distress across cultures. Further, a cutoff of 11 may miss a significant number of women with symptoms below the threshold for major depression, for screening sensitivity is more important that specificity to detect the majority of cases.

In a review of 58 of 83 eligible studies (N = 15,557), 2,069 had major depression. Across studies, a cutoff of 11 led to the highest combined sensitivity and specificity (Levis et al., 2020). Among the studies that used a semi-structured interview (N = 9,066, N = 1,330 with major depression), sensitivity and specificity were 0.85 and 0.84; with a cutoff of 10, they were 0.81 and 0.88; and 0.66 and 0.95 for a cutoff of 13. The higher cutoff dramatically decreased sensitivity but increased specificity. As expected, higher cutoffs identify women with more severe symptoms, but lower cutoffs avoid identifying the highest percentage of women who meet diagnostic criteria. Interestingly, they found no significant difference based on country, but few studies were from low- and middle-income countries.

Dennis et al. (2016) compared cutoffs of 9 vs. 12 using a stratified sample of 1,125 Canadian new mothers who were screened at 1 and 16 weeks postpartum. They found that a cutoff of 9 had greater sensitivity and more accurately identified mothers who were likely to be depressed at 16 weeks. They noted that 64 mothers identified at 1 week with depressive symptoms had recovered by 16 weeks. They found no serious harm in these false positives. The higher cutoff (12/13) led to fewer false positive but was far less sensitive.

High Cutoff: 12 to 14+

A review of 23 studies (N = 5,398) of English-language EPDS found that a cutoff of 13 or higher had a sensitivity 0.8 and a specificity of 0.9 for detecting major depression (O'Connor et al., 2016). A recent random-effects meta-analysis compared the EPDS to the Structured Clinical Interview for DSM (SCID) (Lyubenova et al., 2021). They specifically compared accuracy of EPDS with cutoffs ranging from 9 to 14 to the Structured Clinical Interview-Depression (SCID) (First & Gibbon, 2004). The samples across 29 studies included 7,315 women, 1,017 with SCID scores for major depression. Not surprisingly, a cutoff of 9 yielded a higher percentage of women identified as depressed (28%). In contrast, 22% were depressed with a cutoff of 10, 11% with a cutoff of 13, and 9% with the SCID. The most stringent cutoff—14—identified the same percentage of women as the SCID. The authors concluded that the EPDS did not accurately estimate depression prevalence at lower cutoffs. Then again, they only wanted to measure major depression. If the goal of screening is only to identify major depression, then you must use the higher cutoff. If, however, the goal is to identify all women with symptoms, a lower cutoff is more appropriate.

Variations of the EPDS

As with the Patient Health Questionnaire, researchers have developed shorter versions and began the process by using factor analysis to determine what each item measured.

A sample of 299 women completed the EPDS at 2 to 3 days and 4 to 6 weeks post-partum (Chabrol et al., 2004). As I previously described, the authors extracted three factors: anxiety, depressive mood, and anhedonia. King (2012) found that anxiety symptoms were the only significant ones that predicted postpartum depression at 4 to 6 weeks in her sample of African American women. The anxiety items were self-blame (item 3), anxiety (item 4), scared or panicking (item 5), inability to cope (item 6), and difficulty sleeping (item 7). These studies led to explorations of whether shorter versions were better at identifying depression compared to the full version.

The Edinburgh Postnatal Depression Scale-3 (EPDS-3)

One study used three items of the EPDS—the anxiety subscale—and compared them with the full 10-item scale and the ultra-brief 2-item screener (Kabir et al., 2008). Their sample was 199 14- to 26-year-old participants in an adolescent maternity program. A total of 21% of the mothers met the criteria for depression (EPDS >10). The EPDS-3 had the best performance, with 95% sensitivity and 98% negative predictive value. It identified 16% more mothers as depressed than the full EPDS did. The 3-item screener included the following questions:

- I have blamed myself unnecessarily when things went wrong. (item 3)
- I have been anxious or worried for no good reason. (item 4)
- I have felt scared and panicky for no very good reason. (item 5)

Kabir et al. suggested that the EPDS-3 is brief enough to be incorporated into well-baby checks and identified a higher percentage of women as possibly depressed than the full EPDS.

A study from Western Australia included both antenatal ($N = 4,706$) and postnatal ($N = 3,853$) women and demonstrated the validity of using the EPDS to measure anxiety (Swalm et al., 2010). The items that captured anxiety are numbers 3, 4, and 5. A score of 4 or more on those three items captures the top quartile of mothers at possible high risk for perinatal anxiety disorders.

The Edinburgh Postnatal Depression Scale-2 (EPDS-2)

The 2-item EPDS has not been widely used, largely because of its poor performance and marked inferiority. It resembles the Patient Health Questionnaire-2 (PHQ-2) (see Chapter 4) but is much less effective. It has a sensitivity of 48% and a negative predictive value of 80% (Kabir et al., 2008). These items included the following:

- I have looked forward with enjoyment to things. (item 2)
- I have felt sad or miserable. (item 8)

A study with 249 Black women in South Africa examined the specificity and sensitivity of the full EPDS for prenatal screening compared with shortened versions, including the EPDS-2, 3, 5, and 7 (Hung et al., 2014). The 3-, 5-, and 7-item versions were comparable to the EPDS-10 but all had low sensitivities and specificities. The 2-item version performed even more poorly.

EPDS-US

As this book went to press, a new version of the EPDS appeared in the literature: the Edinburgh Postnatal Depression Scale-United States (EPDS-US) (Moyer et al., 2023). This new version seeks to address limitations of the EPDS with edits to the questions. Their goals are to make the scale sound less judgmental, to eliminate confusing phrases, and to be trauma-informed. For example, they added a new introduction.

> We recognize that there are many different feelings and experiences during pregnancy, birth, postpartum, and parenting. We care about you and we use this form to check-in and as a starting point for conversations.

The authors noted that the language changes reflect both trauma-informed and respectful care guidelines. It also orients the mothers to the purpose of the scale.

- For item 3, the authors removed "unnecessarily" from the question about blaming themselves, feeling that it judged the mother. They also removed "for no good reason" from item 5, which asks about feeling panicky or scared. For item 6, they reworded "things have been getting on top of me" to "I have felt overwhelmed."
- The EPDS question about sleep (item 7) is "I have been so unhappy that I have had difficulty sleeping." This is a poor measure of sleep problems. In our sleep study, many of the mothers had marked sleep issues, yet their experiences were not reflected with this item on the EPDS. I believe that the new version is an improvement. "I have had difficulty sleeping *even when I have the opportunity to sleep.*"
- This scale has not been validated. However, its face validity is good and may address many of the concerns about the EPDS.

EPDS-Partners and EPDS-Lifetime

The EPDS-Partners is a version that detects depression in partners through mothers' report (Fisher et al., 2012). This instrument demonstrated reliability and validity in detecting fathers' depression in a sample of 810 couples. They compared mothers' reports on fathers and the fathers' self-reports. Both types of reports were accurate, although, not surprisingly, fathers' self-reports were somewhat more accurate than mothers' reports about fathers.

Another recent variant is the EPDS-Lifetime, which was modified to include questions about lifetime incidence of postpartum depression, the worst episode, and the timing of symptoms onset. A study using data from the Netherlands Study of Depression and Anxiety evaluated the EPSD-Lifetime (Meltzer-Brody et al., 2013). This study assessed the prevalence of lifetime postpartum depression in women who had histories of prior major depression and evaluated the risk factors for postpartum depression. Fifty-four percent of the women had an episode of major depression before their first episode of postpartum depression. Forty percent of women with a lifetime history of depression and a live birth had an EPDS score >12. Fifty-seven percent happened during postpartum, and 43% occurred during pregnancy. They found that 2 out of 5 parous women with a history of major depression also had postpartum depression. The symptoms of postpartum depression were more severe than those of women in the non-postpartum depression group.

Summary for Optimal Use of the EPDS

In reflecting on the 30 years since the development of the EPDS, Cox (2019), the author of the scale, made recommendations on its optimal use. Users should ensure that they are using it on a population that it has been validated on. Given that the EPDS has been used for populations far beyond its original purpose, this recommendation is reasonable. Cox reminded readers that the EPDS is not a diagnostic tool. It can tell whether depressive symptoms are present, but not their intensity or duration. In addition, the EPDS is not a checklist of common symptoms and does not include somatic symptoms or any measure of the mother–infant relationship. The original purpose of the EPDS was to detect prenatal and postpartum depression in community clinics in Edinburgh, Scotland. If it is used in other countries, it needs to be translated and back-translated. It needs to have face, semantic, conceptual, and technical validity. In this comment, he echoed the concern researchers raised regarding low- to middle-income countries.

He also recommended that health professionals screen with the EPDS and follow up by providing access to mental healthcare. Unfortunately, many consider simply administering the EPDS once to have done due diligence regarding depression, as if it were the intervention rather than a screen. Cox recommended that health professionals discuss mothers' responses with them, listen to their stories, determine if there are other health conditions present, and decide whether they need referral to mental health services or simply need someone to talk to via further "listening sessions."

Clinical Takeaways

- Many programs administer the EPDS because it is so widely used. On a practical note, you might consider whether this scale is appropriate to use with mothers in your community and whether scoring mistakes are likely (e.g., how will they be scored?). The shorter version might better meet your needs.
- Low cutoffs on the EPDS will identify more depressed mothers. Some communities with scarce resources might opt for a more stringent cutoff, allowing them to triage mothers with more severe depressive symptoms.
- The EPDS-3 has good reliability and validity and identifies anxiety symptoms.
- The EPDS-US shows promise and may translate more easily into other cultural's since the English is not colloquial.

4 The Patient Health Questionnaires

The Patient Health Questionnaires (PHQs) are screening tools available for free online, and they are in American English, which is easier for American mothers and may be less colloquial in its phrasing, allowing for easier translation. All versions have good reliability and validity. Three versions stem from the original Patient Health Questionnaire-9 (PHQ-9). The *Diagnostic and Statistical Manual-5* also recommends the PHQ-9 as a tool for evaluating the severity of depression in the general population (Sun et al., 2020). The PHQ scales are widely used in primary care settings to identify depression and anxiety and have been validated for pregnant and postpartum women as well. The three versions that are most widely used are the 9-item PHQ-9, the 2-item PHQ-2, and the 4-item PHQ-4.

KEY FINDINGS

- The PHQs are easy-to-use scales that many prefer to the EPDS because the language is less colloquial. Health organizations also recommend these scales.
- Although designed for a general patient population, the PHQs have been validated for perinatal women.
- The PHQ-4 also assesses anxiety.
- The PHQ-2 has lower reliability and validity compared to the full scale, but many consider its short length an advantage.

Patient Health Questionnaire-9 (PHQ-9)

The master scale, the PHQ-9, is a 9-item multiple-choice inventory. The 9 questions represent the 9 symptoms of major depressive disorder, and it was designed to detect major depression in adults in primary care. It is a self-administered version of the PRIME-MD diagnostic instrument that measures mental disorders and has high specificity and sensitivity. It has also been validated with perinatal patients (Kroenke et al., 2001; Walker et al., 2015). Its major limitation is the lack of an item about suicidal ideation.

Criterion validity was established by comparing it with the results of 580 structured mental health professional interviews. Construct validity was assessed by comparing results with the 20-item Short-Form General Health Survey. It was originally validated on a sample of 6,000 patients: 3,000 from primary care and 3,000 from OB-GYN. The Cronbach's alpha (a measure of internal reliability) was 0.89 for the primary care sample and 0.86 for the OB-GYN sample. It also had excellent test-retest reliability (Kroenke et al., 2001).

DOI: 10.4324/9781003405092-5

One study compared the Patient Health Questionnaire-9 (PHQ-9) and the depression questions from the Pregnancy Risk Assessment Monitoring Systems (PRAMS-6) (Davis et al., 2013). These measures were validated against the Structured Clinical Interview for Depression (SCID) and the Hamilton Depression Rating Scale. The PRAMS-6 and PHQ-9 were both effective for screening for postpartum depression and had moderate accuracy when compared with the SCID. The PHQ-9 had slightly better accuracy than the PRAMS-6.

A study of 745 pregnant women found that the PHQ-9 can also be used during pregnancy (Sidebottom et al., 2012). Patients were assessed in early pregnancy with the PHQ-9. During later pregnancy, mothers were assessed via clinical interview. The PHQ-9 had good sensitivity (85%) and specificity (84%) and accurately identified depression in pregnant women.

Patient Health Questionnaire-2 (PHQ-2)

The 2-item Patient Health Questionnaire (PHQ-2) is a shortened version of the PHQ-9, which can be used in all healthcare settings. It has also been validated to use with new mothers (Walker et al., 2015), and both the American Academy of Pediatrics and the American College of Obstetricians and Gynecologists recommend its use (Earls & The Committee on Psychosocial Aspects of Child and Family Health, 2010). However, if results on the PHQ-2 are positive for depression (a score more than 3), they recommend assessing mothers with the full PHQ-9.

The PHQ-2 assesses frequency of anhedonia ("little interest or pleasure in doing things") and depressed mood ("feeling down, depressed, or hopeless") during the past two weeks.

Over the past two weeks, how often have you been bothered by any of the following problems?

- Little interest or pleasure in doing things
- Feeling down, depressed, or hopeless

The response categories include "Not at All," "Several Days," "More Than Half the Days," and "Nearly Every Day" and are scored from 0 to 3. A score over 3 indicates possible depression.

One study found that the PHQ-2 was highly sensitive for identifying postpartum depression during well-child visits (Gjerdingen et al., 2009). However, another study found that the PHQ-2 was not effective in identifying depression in low-income women (Cutler et al., 2007). Ninety-four women participated in this study from an inner-city well-child clinic. There was moderate agreement between PHQ-2 and EPDS. The sensitivity of the PHQ-2 was 44%, and specificity 93%. The sensitivity was higher for mothers with more education. In other words, it was not detecting depression in low-income, low-education mothers, a group that is at higher risk. Clinicians working with mothers in these populations should be aware that this is a weakness of the scale.

A study of postpartum women from Kenya found that the PHQ-2 did not detect depression as well as other measures (Larsen et al., 2023). This study included 3,605 women and compared the prevalence of moderate to severe depression using the Center for Epidemiologic Studies Depression Scale (CESD-10), the Edinburgh Postnatal

Depression Scale (EPDS), and the Patient Health Questionnaire-9 and 2 (PHQ-9 and PHQ-2). The PHQ-2 detected the smallest percentage of depressed women compared to the other scales.

Another study compared the Edinburgh Postnatal Depression Scale to the PHQ-2 for their accuracy in detecting depression in 252 pregnant women from Australia (Slavin et al., 2020). They also found that the PHQ-2 had low sensitivity (i.e., failed to detect women who were depressed) but high specificity using cutoffs of both 2 or 3. They tested women at 4 points during pregnancy and postpartum. They concluded that the PHQ-2 missed an unacceptably high number of women with major depression. One possible reason is that the PHQ-2 does not include questions about anxiety, which the authors of the EPDS-3 discovered were critical. The PHQ-4 addresses this limitation.

Patient Health Questionnaire-4 (PHQ-4)

The PHQ-4 is an ultra-brief measure that combines the PHQ-2 with the GAD-2 (The Generalized Anxiety Disorder-2 Scale), a 2-item anxiety scale (Kroenke et al., 2009). The scale accurately predicts generalized anxiety disorder, panic disorder, and social anxiety disorder, but not posttraumatic stress disorder.

A German study of 5,030 men and women tested the construct validity of the PHQ-2 and 4 and the GAD-2 (Lowe et al., 2010). The study supported the reliability and validity of the PHQ-4, PHQ-2, and GAD-2 as measures of depression and anxiety in the general population. A study with data collected in 2020 (N = 2,503) and 2021 (N = 2,519) provided continued support for the PHQ-2, PHQ-4, and GAD-2 (Wicke et al., 2022).

A study of 6,874 women who had given birth in the past 6 months explored mothers' health after giving birth during the COVID-19 pandemic (Basu et al., 2021). These women were from 64 countries. To measure anxiety and depression, they used the PHQ-4. They noted that the depression items were drawn from the PHQ-8, and the anxiety items from the General Anxiety Disorders-7. The results from the PHQ-4 yielded results consistent with the measures of PTSD and worry (i.e., anxiety and depression correlated with worry and PTSD). The PHQ-4 indicated that 31% exceeded the threshold for depression or anxiety.

The most recent Listening to Mothers in California survey (N = 2,539), a representative sample based on birth certificates, also used the PHQ-4 to measure depression and anxiety (Declercq et al., 2021). The authors found that the PHQ-4 was a valid measure for all the mothers in their study, including racial/ethnic minorities. Finally, the PHQ-4 was used to measure depression and anxiety in an 11-year longitudinal study of 20 women who developed pregnancy and lactation-related osteoporosis (Gehlen et al., 2019).

A Spanish study tested the psychometric properties and validation of the PHQ-4 for pregnant women (Rodriguez-Munoz et al., 2020). The study included 845 pregnant women recruited from public hospitals. Exploratory and confirmatory factor analysis and intercorrelations between the PHQ-9 and PHQ-4 found that the PHQ-4 adequately assessed depression and anxiety during pregnancy. They concluded that it was a reliable and valid instrument for use with pregnant women.

A study from rural Pakistan used three short screening tools to screen for depression and anxiety: the PHQ-4, the 4-item Hamilton Depression Rating Scale, and the Community Informant Detection Tool (Waqas et al., 2021). All were effective. They found that the PHQ-4 had "excellent psychometric properties to screen for perinatal depression," with a sensitivity of 93.4% and specificity of 91.7%.

Another recent study examined the reliability and validity of the PHQ-4 for pregnant women (Barrera et al., 2021). Their sample included 1,148 pregnant women of diverse cultural background who were English ($N = 587$) or Spanish ($N = 561$) speaking. Using confirmatory factor analysis, they found that the PHQ-4 showed good reliability and validity for pregnant women as a screen for anxiety and depression. They noted, however, that to make a diagnosis, clinicians need to follow the initial screen with a clinical interview.

The PHQ-4 uses the same two questions as on the PHQ-2 but adds two anxiety questions:

- Feeling nervous, anxious, or on edge
- Not being able to control or stop worrying

The PHQ-4 uses the same response categories as the PHQ-2. A score of 3 or more on the first two questions suggests anxiety, and a score of 3 or more on the PHQ-2 (questions 3 and 4) suggests depression (Wicke et al., 2022).

Overall, I prefer the PHQ-4 to the EPDS, but both are effective in clinical settings, and both are useful in research. One limitation is that the Patient Health Questionnaires are designed to screen for depression in the general population and might miss some important nuances with postpartum mental illness.

Clinical Takeaways

- The PHQs are excellent choices for screening perinatal women. However, no scale is perfect and should be matched to the needs of your community.
- The scales with the highest reliability are the PHQ-9 and the PHQ-4. The PHQ-2 is useful, but its reliability and validity are lower.
- The PHQ-4 also includes a brief measure for anxiety adapted from the Generalized Anxiety Disorders-2 Scale.

5 Other Screening Tools

In addition to the Patient Health Questionnaires and the Edinburgh Postnatal Depression Scale, there are other measures that may prove useful for both practitioners and researchers. These scales measure depression, PTSD, sleep, birth trauma, and bipolar disorder.

KEY FINDINGS

- Scales in this chapter assess depression, PTSD, birth trauma, maternal sleep, and bipolar disorder.
- While all these scales provide useful information, only two are specific to perinatal women, so the results of the other scales must be interpreted with caution (e.g., normal postpartum sleep may appear pathological on a scale designed to measure sleep problems in the general population).

The Postpartum Depression Screening Scale

The Postpartum Depression Screening Scale (PDSS) is another tool designed specifically for new mothers, which uses DSM-IV criteria for depression (Beck & Gable, 2000). The PDSS is a 35-item, Likert scale, self-report instrument. It measures functioning on seven dimensions: sleeping/eating disturbances, anxiety/insecurity, emotional lability, cognitive impairment, loss of self, guilt/shame, and contemplating harming oneself. It takes 5 to 10 minutes to complete and is available for a small fee from Western Psychological Services (www.wpspublish.com). A shorter 7-item version of this scale has been validated for use with postpartum women (Walker et al., 2015). In a large collaborative trial, midwives and obstetricians were willing to use it (Mancini et al., 2007).

Like the EPDS, the PDSS is designed to screen for postpartum depression. The subscales highlight specific areas of difficulty. In developing this scale, Beck and Gable (2000) attempted to address the limitations of the EPDS. For example, they noted that the EPDS did not measure postpartum feelings, such as loss of control, loneliness, irritability, fear of going crazy, obsessive thinking, concentration difficulties, and loss of self. In a study of 525 new mothers, confirmatory factor analysis supported the seven dimensions of the PDSS. The internal consistencies on the seven dimensions ranged from 0.83 (sleeping/eating disturbances) to 0.94 (loss of self) (Appels et al., 2000).

The Postpartum Depression Screening Scale and the Beck Depression Inventory-II were compared to results of the Structured Clinical Interview-Depression (SCID) with a diverse group of 238 mothers of infants 4 to 15 months old. The goal was to detect major depression beyond the postpartum period (Vogeli et al., 2018). The sample was

DOI: 10.4324/9781003405092-6

68% White, 17% Latina, 9% Black, and 1% Native American. The PDSS subscales were highly accurate. Sensitivity and specificity for major depression were comparable to the Beck Depression Inventory-II (BDI-II). Accuracy was the same across ethnicities.

A confirmatory factor analysis indicated that five factors fit the data better than the original seven identified by Beck and Gable (2000). They include sleeping/eating disturbance, anxiety/insecurity/emotional lability/mental confusion, loss of self/guilt/shame, and suicidal thoughts (Vogeli et al., 2018). The scale had high internal consistency ($\alpha = 0.95$), but the suicidal thoughts subscale was lower than the 0.70 cutoff. The PDSS correctly identified 83% of non-depressed mothers as not depressed and 81% of depressed mothers as depressed. The BDI-II only correctly identified 75% of depressed mothers. The specificity was 0.83, and sensitivity was 0.83.

In a study from Portugal, 503 pregnant women were interviewed and completed the Portuguese versions of the Postpartum Depression Screening Scale and the Beck Depression Inventory-II (Pereira et al., 2011). They found that the PDSS was accurate in detecting depression in pregnant women, with a sensitivity and specificity higher than 80%. They felt that it had an advantage over the BDI-II in that it was specific to motherhood.

A Chinese study used both the EPDS and PDSS with a sample of 842 women with pregnancy complications (Zhao et al., 2015). The EPDS and PDSS both did well in detecting both major and minor depression. But the PDSS performed better psychometrically than the EPDS. Ten percent of women had an EPDS score of 13 or more, and 31% had an EPDS score of 9 to 12. When both scales were used together, the authors recommended a cutoff of 8/9 on the EPDS, with 72% sensitivity and 88% specificity. The cutoff recommended on the PDSS was 79/80 for major depression, with sensitivity of 86% and specificity of 100%. However, the PDSS missed some cases of depression. The authors concluded that both tools were reliable for assessing Chinese pregnant women with complications and recommended using lower cutoffs to reduce misdiagnosis and improve validity of screening. They recommended using both screening tools together and to screen pregnant women at the first prenatal visit.

A study of 123 women compared the accuracy of three scales: Edinburgh Postnatal Depression Scale (EPDS), the PHQ-9, and the PDSS-short version, a 7-item scale (Hanusa et al., 2008). Using DSM-IV criteria for major depression, they found that the EPDS (cutoff >10) detected 62% of cases, the PHQ-9 (cutoff >10) identified 31%, and the PDSS-SF (cutoff >14) identified 92%. However, 94% without depression also screened positive. They found that the EPDS and PDSS-SF were significantly more accurate than the PHQ-9. However, their findings may have been due to the small number of women identified as depressed ($N = 13$).

The City Birth Trauma Scale

The City Birth Trauma Scale is a 29-item measure designed to assess birth-related PTSD (Ayers et al., 2018). It is the first scale that measures birth trauma with the DSM-5 criteria for trauma, including the stressor criteria, and symptoms of re-experiencing, avoidance, negative cognitions and mood, and hyperarousal. However, the authors also added DSM-IV criteria for criterion A: that women responded to their births with fear, helplessness, and horror. It has good reliability (Cronbach's $\alpha = 0.92$) and validity.

The French version of this scale established both the reliability and validity of this measure (Sandoz et al., 2022). The German version showed convergent validity with the

Impact of Events Scale-Revised (IES-R) and the PTSD Check List-5 (PCL-5) (Weigl et al., 2021). It has been validated in Spain with a sample of 207 mothers (Caparros-Gonzalez et al., 2021), and in Brazil with 343 new mothers, it had a sensitivity of 72% and specificity of 83% (Osorio et al., 2022). The Swedish version also had high internal consistency and good test-retest reliability with a sample of 619 women at 6 to 16 weeks. The prevalence of birth trauma was 3.8% (Sten et al., 2023).

A cross-sectional study of 603 women completed the City Birth Trauma Scale, Impact of Events Scale-Revised, the Edinburgh Postnatal Depression Scale, and the anxiety subscale of the Depression, Anxiety, and Stress Scale (DASS-21) (Rados et al., 2020). They found that convergent and divergent validity were high, especially for birth trauma symptoms. They found high discriminant validity for the birth-related symptoms compared to the general symptoms.

However, even though this scale is widely used, there are some methodological concerns. DSM-5 Criterion A of the PTSD diagnosis defines events that rise to sufficient severity to be called "traumatic events." The Criterion A events in the DSM-5 include actual or threatened death, actual or threatened serious injury, and actual or threatened sexual violation. In the older DSM-IV criteria, there were similar criteria, *and* the person had to respond to these events with "fear, helplessness, or horror." In DSM-5, "fear," "helplessness," and "horror" were deleted from Criterion A but are listed among the other symptoms. In other words, you do not *have to* respond with fear, helplessness, or horror, but you *can*. Making "fear, helplessness, and horror" a requirement lowers the number of people diagnosed with PTSD. Ayers, the author of the CBTI, also noted that when she uses the DSM-IV criteria, the incidence of PTSD decreases by 2%. Since the incidence in her studies is typically 4% to 5%, 2% is substantial.

Another concern has to do with questions concerning what happened (Ayers et al., 2018). The CBTI asks, "Did you believe you or your baby would be seriously injured" and "Did you believe you or your baby would die?" The scale does not ask about sexual violation (1 of the 3 possible traumatic events in DSM criteria). Given the number of women in qualitative studies who describe their births as rapes, not asking about it might also underestimate incidence.

Partner Version of the City Birth Trauma Scale

The City Birth Trauma Scale has also been developed for partners who witness traumatic birth (Webb et al., 2021). The scale is also 29 items and has the same factor structure: stressor criteria (A), symptoms of re-experiencing (B), avoidance (C), negative cognitions and mood (D), hyperarousal (E), duration of symptoms (F), and significant distress or impairment. They also added the A2 criteria from DSM-IV about fear, helplessness, and horror. The sample was 301 fathers or partners.

Factor analysis found birth-related and general symptoms. In the validation sample, 60% reported a preterm birth, with the average gestational age of 34 weeks, and 4% reported that their infants had died. Twenty-two percent of fathers or partners met criteria for PTSD, and these symptoms caused a lot of distress. The scale had good reliability and validity. This percentage is higher than it was for mothers, but they advertised and recruited their sample through a birth trauma organization and an organization for parents of preemies, inadvertently recruiting a high-risk sample.

Findings on partners' vs mothers' responses is interesting. Partners reported more medical emergencies than you see in the literature for birth trauma in mothers. Samples of mothers with infants in the neonatal intensive care unit (NICU) show comparable rates of PTSD. In general birth trauma studies, however, women are more likely to report subjective aspects of their births, such as how providers treat them rather than medical emergencies (Simpson & Catling, 2016).

Patient Checklist for PTSD-DSM-5 (PCL-5)

The PCL-5 is a 20-item self-report measure of PTSD. It is available from the US National Center for PTSD and corresponds to the DSM-5 criteria for posttraumatic stress disorder in the general population. The PCL-5 is not specific to perinatal women, but it can screen for and monitor symptoms (Weathers et al., 2013). Severity scores can range from 0 to 80. A cutoff of 31 to 33 indicates probable PTSD. The gold standard for PTSD diagnosis is the Clinician-Administered PTSD Scale (CAPS-5), but the PCL-5 can provide a provisional diagnosis.

The psychometric properties of the PCL-5 were examined in two studies of trauma-exposed college students (Blevins et al., 2015). The first study included 278 students. They were 71% White and 12% Black. There was strong internal consistency ($\alpha = .94$), with good test-retest reliability, and convergent and discriminant validity. There was adequate fit with a confirmatory factor analysis with the DSM-5 4-factor model. The second study, with 558 students, had similar reliability and validity. In this sample, 86% were White and 8% were Black. The City Birth Trauma Scale was validated against the PCL-5 (Weigl et al., 2021). The PCL-5 has also been used along with the EPDS and the City Birth Trauma Scale to assess PTSD following childbirth in a sample of 980 participants in an online study of birth trauma (Ertan et al., 2021).

Pittsburgh Sleep Quality Index (PSQI)

The Pittsburgh Sleep Quality Index (PSQI) is a 9-item scale that asks about a person's sleep over the past month. It assesses seven domains of sleep and is widely used worldwide (Buysse et al., 1989). It was not developed for postpartum women, so it does not account for baby-related waking or the impact of feeding method on sleep. However, it can provide useful information about a mother's overall functioning. A meta-analysis of 37 studies found good reliability and validity, though quality of the studies varied (Mollayeva et al., 2016).

The PSQI was validated with a sample of 1,488 pregnant women (Qui et al., 2016). Researchers used a structured interview to collect data regarding sleep and demographic factors. They also used the PHQ-9 and the Depression, Anxiety, and Stress Scale-21 (DASS-21) to assess depression, anxiety, and stress. The PSQI positively correlated with the PHQ-9 and DASS-21, demonstrating good construct validity, and the reliability was 0.74. The authors concluded that the PSQI was a reliable and valid scale for assessing sleep in pregnant women.

A recent meta-analysis of 42 studies examined sleep quality in perinatal and postnatal women using the PSQI (Yang et al., 2020). The prevalence of poor sleep was 54% and 67% for postnatal women. Interestingly, poor sleep varied by region: North America, 75%; Asia, 54%; and Europe, 51%. Not surprisingly, a lower cutoff on the PSQI yielded a higher prevalence than a higher cutoff.

When assessing fatigue and sleep, Preston et al. (2022) recommend also asking about caffeine use. They noted that using caffeine more than 250 milligrams per day can decrease slow-wave sleep, which worsens depression. (A cup of coffee has 125 milligrams.) Caffeine is also related to frequent wakings and restless sleep. Insomnia can occur even when people do not have trouble going to sleep. They noted that patients do not generally take caffeine intake seriously until a healthcare provider explains its impact on sleep.

The Mood Disorder Questionnaire (MDQ)

The Mood Disorder Questionnaire is a 13-item measure of possible bipolar disorder, which the EPDS and PHQ-9 do not assess (Hirschfeld et al., 2000). As bipolar disorder is the underlying condition most associated with postpartum psychosis, identifying it quickly can prevent a tragedy. Clark and Wisner (2018) advise using the EPDS, PHQ-9, and the MDQ before beginning pharmacotherapy. Bipolar disorder can initially present as major depressive disorder until antidepressants trigger a manic episode. Before prescribing an antidepressant, it is helpful to rule out possible bipolar disorder.

The sensitivity and specificity of the Mood Disorder Questionnaire was assessed for 150 women who were referred for psychiatric assessment during pregnancy ($N = 95$) or postpartum ($N = 55$) (Frey et al., 2012). Eighteen women (12%) were diagnosed with bipolar disorder (6 with bipolar I, 10 with bipolar II). Using a cutoff of 7, they found that sensitivity was 89% and specificity was 84%. Given that 25% of women with bipolar disorder relapse during pregnancy and half relapse postpartum, assessment and monitoring are essential. In addition, the MDQ can also identify new cases, which is especially pertinent before antidepressants are administered.

A study compared 57 postpartum women with bipolar disorder to 68 women with postpartum major depression (Sharma & Xie, 2011). Using an optimal cutoff of 8, they found a sensitivity of 88% and specificity of 85%. The specificity and sensitivity were lower with traditional scoring. The authors concluded that the MSQ was a useful tool for screening for bipolar disorder in the postpartum period.

Clinical Takeaways

- All scales in this chapter can provide useful information. However, mothers may find completing several questionnaires onerous and refuse to do it. Shorter screening tools do not provide as much information, but *some* may be preferable to *none* if mothers refuse to complete longer forms.
- When contemplating which scales to use, consider the needs and limitations of your program. Will you be able to address the issues you assess? Do you have resources available for someone with sleep disorders, PTSD, or bipolar disorder? Will you use these scales for every mother or only for those with symptoms?

6 Assessing for Symptom Severity, Maternal Suicide Risk, and Possible Infant Harm

Once a mother screens positive for depression, it is important to determine the severity of her symptoms. It is also important to screen for risk of maternal suicide or possible infant harm. Other considerations are whether she is abusing substances or requires hospitalization. If you are part of a community organization that has screened for depression, this next section may not be within your scope of practice. However, mothers who have screened positive will need to be referred for this type of evaluation.

KEY FINDINGS

- The first marker of severity will be mothers' score on an assessment tool. Severity can also be determined through patient and family members' report.
- Symptoms of suicide risk include a previous history of suicide attempts, specific suicide plans, and conditions such as substance use or personality disorder. Mothers who are isolated are more at risk. But all mothers with depression, anxiety, or PTSD should be assessed.
- Obsessive-compulsive thoughts of infant harm do not mean a mother is at risk for harming her infant. Mothers with these thoughts will often go to great lengths to prevent bad things from happening. In contrast, concerning thoughts of infant harm are those that are consistent with mothers' beliefs (e.g., believing that their infants are demon-possessed). It is important to differentiate between the two.

Severity of the Current Episode

Three factors contribute to the severity of depression: duration and intensity of symptoms and level of impairment. To diagnose major depression, symptoms must be present for at least 2 weeks. Severe symptoms and impairment suggest that aggressive treatment is warranted. When mothers are severely impaired, they may stop bathing, may not be able to manage their household, or may have days when they cannot get out of bed. If symptoms are serious enough, they might need to be hospitalized. Ideally, their infants can accompany them.

Moses-Kolko and Roth (2004) recommend a full psychiatric evaluation if a woman scores above 9 on the EPDS. If a full psychological evaluation is not an option, you can triage mothers who need immediate assistance.

1. Is she thinking of harming herself or her baby?
2. Do other members of her family have a psychiatric history?

DOI: 10.4324/9781003405092-7

3. What is her gravid and psychosocial history?
4. What do her lab results (including TSH) indicate?
5. Does she have symptoms or a family history of bipolar disorder?

If symptoms persist for more than 2 weeks, she should be referred for treatment.

A woman who scores between 5 and 9 on the EPDS may be at risk for depression within the next 6 to 12 months. Clinicians can give women copies of the EPDS and instruct them to seek care if they score 9 or above. If they intend to harm themselves or their babies, they should be seen immediately (Moses-Kolko & Roth, 2004). A woman with a EPDS score <5 is unlikely to be depressed and needs no further follow-up.

If mothers are hospitalized while still breastfeeding and they want to continue, they will need a hospital-grade pump to prevent mastitis, plugged ducts, and infection, and to protect their milk supply. When mothers can provide their milk, it makes them feel connected to their babies. Pumping milk also gives mothers a vision of life beyond the hospital. If mothers choose to wean, it should be gradual, as sudden weaning increases their risk of mastitis and possible infection.

Suicide Risk

Although rare, maternal suicide is so serious that all depressed mothers should be screened. The Institute for Clinical Systems Improvement (Nicolson et al., 2013) lists specific risk factors for suicide. Be sure to chart your assessment of suicide risk, and do not be afraid to screen as often as you think necessary. Does she have:

- A previous history of suicide attempts;
- Suicidal ideation, particularly with specific suicide plans;
- Substance abuse or dependency;
- A personality disorder or physical illness; or
- A family history of suicide?

Is she:

- Single,
- Recently bereaved, or
- Recently divorced or separated?

Does she have:

- Insomnia,
- Panic attacks,
- Diminished concentration,
- Severe anhedonia or hopelessness, or
- Comorbid PTSD?

Another red-flag symptom is insomnia that has persisted for 2 or more days. No sleep for 2 or 3 days is often a prodrome to postpartum psychosis.

If even one of these risk factors is present, a more specialized consult is in order. Potentially suicidal patients should be closely monitored through frequent visits, by residing with family or friends, or by being hospitalized. Contact your local suicide prevention hotline for information about how best to proceed, and for referrals of people in your community who can help.

Possible Infant Harm

Infant safety must always be a top concern, but it is important to distinguish between mothers' thoughts of infant harm related to obsessive-compulsive disorder and delusions where she is at risk for harming her baby (Williams & Koleva, 2018). In a systematic review, mothers had obsessive thoughts about accidentally harming their babies that were common. These included checking compulsions, self-reassurance, and seeking reassurance from others (Starcevic et al., 2020). Other types of obsessive thoughts concerned their babies dying in their sleep, or that they would sexually abuse or physically misplace them. Not surprisingly, obsessive thoughts can be very troubling to mothers. This mother describes how she developed symptoms of obsessive-compulsive disorder (OCD) and panic disorder after a previous stillbirth and high-risk pregnancy. Her symptoms started at 6 months postpartum.

> I was nervous about everything. About germs, development, baby care, all of it. I started having these thoughts about Zeke's safety. The scariest part were these weird thoughts about harming him myself. I was afraid to say anything to anybody. They terrified me. I kept hoping it would go away. It didn't. . . .
>
> My husband had an Employee Assistance Program that was also available to spouses. I didn't know where else to go, but I called them the next day when nobody else was there. I used a quiet voice and felt huge shame. . . . They got me set up with a counselor in my area who diagnosed me with postpartum depression. . . .
>
> That next counselor was a godsend. She talked to me about my expectations, reassured me that I wouldn't hurt my baby, and helped me know when it was time for antidepressants. I slowly got better.

Speisman et al. (2011) noted that psychotic symptoms are not present in OCD. In psychosis, mothers' thoughts of harming their infants are consistent with their delusional thinking. A person acts out aggressive behavior or because she believes she must do it (e.g., she believes her baby is possessed by the devil). In contrast, mothers' obsessive thoughts about infant harm *do not* increase the risk that they will act on them. These thoughts are unwanted and inconsistent with a person's normal behavior and are so distressing that people will go to great lengths to keep bad things from happening.

When speaking to a mother, say something like this: "It must be very distressing to you to have such thoughts. Many other women have these thoughts, and they do not mean that you are a bad mother or will harm your baby. These thoughts usually mean that you are experiencing severe stress, and it may help to talk with someone about it." This type of approach validates her experience while taking the problem seriously.

Unfortunately, there are times when you may need to take more drastic action. If you fear that the baby is in danger, you may be legally obligated to make a report to the department of social services or your local child protective agency. But in most cases, that will not be necessary.

Clinical Takeaways

- Assessing for possible maternal or infant harm is more subjective than using a scale. However, there are conditions and symptoms that indicate increased risk.
- Be sure to chart all interactions you have with mothers around these topics.
- If you are concerned, get a specialized assessment. While we do not want to overreact, the stakes are so high that getting another assessment, and making sure that mothers have extra support, is prudent.

Section II

Complementary and Integrative Treatments

7 An Integrative Approach to Treatment

Once identified, postpartum depression needs to be treated promptly. For many decades, the frontline treatment was antidepressants, with possible psychotherapy as an afterthought. Fortunately, there are now many other effective options. The following sections describe the full range of treatments that practitioners have used in countries around the world. Some treatments have a strong evidence base; others are newer and have less of one. In each section, I summarize the available evidence so that you can make informed decisions. I encourage you to think creatively about how you can tap into resources available in your community. The more options mothers have, the more willing they may to seek treatment for their symptoms.

KEY FINDINGS

- There is a wide range of treatment choices available beyond medications and psychotherapy. You have many opportunities to help families find the type of treatment they are most comfortable with.
- Mothers may choose complementary and alternative (CAM) treatments for a variety of reasons. Many CAM treatments are as effective as medications and can be safely tried.
- It is important to reassess mothers 4 to 6 weeks after treatment begins to ensure that their symptoms are improving. This is also true for medications. Unfortunately, most mothers are never evaluated again once treatment starts, and they may still be depressed.

Mothers' Acceptance of Treatment

Your treatment may be the best in the world, but if mothers refuse, it will not do any good. White middle-class mothers were among the first who were identified as having postpartum depression. Our treatment approaches have been shaped by this demographic reality. They were all prescribed medications and told to wean. A few had psychotherapy.

Clinicians make a mistake when they assume that this treatment approach works for everyone. Many mothers either have no access to that type of treatment or they don't want it. If medications are the only options on the table, mothers may avoid treatment altogether—and they are still depressed. Some cultures do not accept antidepressants because they distrust Western healthcare. Not surprisingly, these mothers look for alternatives. In one study, more than half of the participants used alternative treatments to treat depression and anxiety (Werneke et al., 2006).

DOI: 10.4324/9781003405092-9

A systematic review of 35 articles focused on women's use of mental health services and their predisposition toward them (Bina, 2020). One factor is women's perceived need for treatment. Women's immigration status and the norms in their community can impact their decision about seeking treatment. Unfortunately, relatively few depressed women seek treatment, even after screening (Bina, 2020).

Complementary and Alternative Treatments for Depression

Any approach that does not use medication could be called "complementary and alternative" (CAM). Technically, this definition can also include social support interventions and psychotherapy, but most practitioners describe them separately. Most CAM modalities can be combined or used with medications (Miller, 2008). For example, long-chain omega-3 fatty acids boast the effectiveness of antidepressants. Exercise can be combined with social support and bright light therapy. The American Psychiatric Association noted that effective CAM treatments could expand the "toolbox" of possible treatments and possibly engage more patients (Freeman et al., 2010).

From the patient's perspective, using non-drug treatments offers several advantages. Women often prefer these modalities because they are concerned about control, privacy, costs, and safety.

- **Control.** With CAM, patients can control their own healthcare. Instead of having to wait for a provider, they can start treatment right away.
- **Privacy.** Patients may be ashamed to admit that they are depressed and are frightened about others finding out. A prescription for antidepressants increases their vulnerability of exposure. Unfortunately, medication information sometimes *does* get released, even with confidentiality regulations in place. Patients may want to avoid that possibility and treat themselves.
- **Costs.** Newer antidepressants can be expensive. For patients without insurance, the cost can be prohibitive. In contrast, many CAM modalities are reasonably priced. The savings can be substantial.
- **Side Effects and Safety.** Side effect and safety profiles of CAM modalities are usually better than those for medications (Freeman et al., 2010; Klier et al., 2006; Schultz, 2006). Patients often stop taking antidepressants because they do not like the side effects (Preston et al., 2022). In addition, many women fear possible teratogenic effects of medications taken during pregnancy and breastfeeding and therefore may be reluctant to take antidepressants at all (Dennis & Allen, 2008). (See Chapter 20.)

Do Non-Drug Treatments Work?

The short answer is "yes." Understandably, some practitioners will not support using these modalities without an evidence base. The American Psychiatric Association's Task Force on Complementary and Alternative Medicine in Major Depressive Disorder urged caution and balanced consideration in the use of CAM therapies (Freeman et al., 2010). They recommended weighing each CAM treatment based on scientific evidence regarding its safety and efficacy. Practitioners should monitor all patients with depression for efficacy of treatment, side effects, and possible worsening of symptoms.

An integrative approach to treatment combines medical care with evidence-based complementary and alternative modalities. These options can be tailored to individual mothers. The rest of this book provides an overview of treatments that work, across the spectrum, using an integrative approach.

In the following chapters, I describe CAM treatments, social support, psychotherapy, and medications. As you evaluate these treatments, keep in mind that even generally effective treatments do not work for every mother. Therefore, it is important to assess mothers periodically (e.g., every month or so) to see if their symptoms have remitted. If they have not, another treatment can be tried or added.

We begin with nutraceuticals. *Nutraceuticals* are nutritional supplements that have a physiological benefit. A *dietary supplement* is a vitamin or mineral, an amino acid, a medical herb, or a concentrate, metabolite, constituent, extract, or combinations of these ingredients. The nutraceuticals I describe in the next two chapters include long-chain omega-3 fatty acids, vitamins D and B-12, curcumin, and St. John's wort.

Clinical Takeaways

- Many complementary and alternative treatments have evidence that supports their use.
- Mothers may opt for these approaches because they do not want to take medications. Other reasons include cost, their privacy, and side effects. Some of these approaches may also be more acceptable in their communities.
- As is true with all treatments, re-assessing mothers at 4 to 6 weeks is important to determine if their symptoms are improving. If not, a different approach should be tried.

8 Nutraceuticals I
Long-Chain Omega-3 Fatty Acids

Over the past 150 years, the diets in Western populations made a critical shift, specifically in the ratio of omega-6 to omega-3 fatty acids, which has had a negative impact on our health. As a population, we have decreased the amount of anti-inflammatory omega-3s we consume while increasing our consumption of proinflammatory omega-6s. Omega-6s are common in many vegetable oils and therefore are also found in almost all processed foods. Many of the snack items we enjoy raise our inflammation levels. At the same time, we avoid foods with fats that lower inflammation.

KEY FINDINGS

- The long-chain omega-3 EPA is the only omega-3 that treats depression. However, the findings have been mixed, and there is some controversy about the correct dosage (1 vs. 2 grams).
- DHA does not treat depression but can prevent it. It also prevents preterm birth.
- The safest sources of EPA and DHA are fish oil capsules verified to be free of contaminants. There are many cost-effective choices available.

Omega-6s and omega-3s are both part of a category called "polyunsaturated fatty acids" (PUFAs), which means that they are liquid at room temperature (see Figure 8.1). Omega-3s and 6s are essential fatty acids, which means that we need to consume them— We cannot make them. While some omega-6s are necessary for good nutrition, they become harmful when the ratio of omega-6s to omega-3s is too high—as it is in modern diets. Kiecolt-Glaser and colleagues (2007) noted that the hunter–gatherer diet had an estimated ratio of omega-6s to omega-3s of 2:1 or 3:1. In contrast, the typical North American diet, with its high amounts of vegetable oils in processed foods, ranges from 15:1 to 17:1. There is a similar pattern in Australia and New Zealand, with a ratio approximately 10:1 (Rees et al., 2005).

Regarding depression, the long-chain omega-3s are of interest. These are eicosapentaenoic acid (EPA) and docosahexaenoic acid (DHA). Alpha-linolenic acid (ALA) is the parent omega-3 fatty acid and is found in flaxseed, nuts, and other plant sources (see Figure 8.1). While ALA is important for good nutrition, it is too metabolically removed from the long-chain omega-3s to be sufficiently anti-inflammatory and cannot prevent or treat of depression (Freeman et al., 2006a). Only about 10% of ALA that we consume is metabolized into long-chain omega-3s.

People who are depressed often have lower concentrations of omega-3s, which changes the ratio between EPA and ARA in cell membranes. ARA is arachidonic acid, a

DOI: 10.4324/9781003405092-10

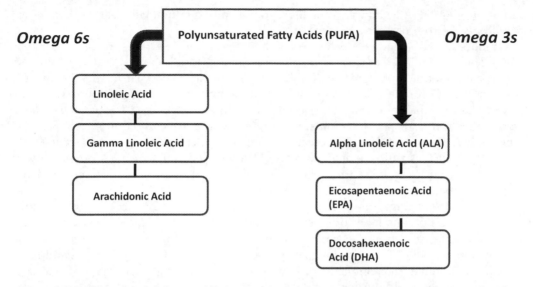

Figure 8.1 Polyunsaturated fatty acids: omega-6s and omega-3s. Boxes across from each other reflect using the same metabolic pathways. Open access.

Source: (Wang et al., 2004).

long-chain omega-6 that increases inflammation. Patients with higher arachidonic acid were more likely to be depressed (Rechenberg & Humphries, 2013). Low levels of anti-inflammatory omega-3s change the fluidity and structure of the brain, which change the metabolism of neurotransmitters, such as serotonin-norepinephrine and dopamine. These neurotransmitters influence mental health.

Omega-3s and Depression in Population Studies

Much of the research on the mental health effects of omega-3s comes from studying population-level fish consumption. People who eat a lot of fish have lower rates of mood and anxiety disorders, including perinatal depression. The amount of fish necessary to achieve these protective effects was about 50 pounds of seafood a year (1 to 1.5 pounds per person per week) (Noaghiul & Hibbeln, 2003).

Hibbeln (2002) found that postpartum depression was up to 50 times more common in countries with low fish consumption in his study of 14,000 women in 22 countries. For example, the rate of postpartum depression in Singapore was 0.5%, compared to 24.5% in South Africa. Similarly, Rees and colleagues (2005) observed that the rates for post-partum depression in North America and Europe are 10 times those in Taiwan, Japan, Hong Kong, and some regions of China. A study of 55 women from Western Norway found that lower levels of EPA/DHA at 28 weeks' gestation predicted higher levels of depression at 3 months postpartum (Markhus et al., 2013). Norway has high rates of fish consumption.

In contrast, a study of 865 pregnant women in Japan did not find lower rates of depression in women who ate more fish (Miyake et al., 2006). This may be a ceiling effect; because Japan has one of the highest rates of fish consumption in the world. In addition, EPA/DHA levels were estimated from dietary questionnaires rather than measured directly from participant plasma.

A more recent Japanese study had similar findings in a prospective study of 967 women after delivery and 710 women at 6 months postpartum (Kobayashi et al., 2017). EPA and DHA consumption in late pregnancy did not lower the risk of postpartum depression at 1 or 6 months. A couple of factors might explain their findings. Since everyone had a high level, "higher" may not have made a difference. In addition, as in the previous study, fatty acids were calculated via dietary questionnaires, not measured in serum. Second, they only measured intake in late pregnancy and yet expected a carryover effect at 1 and 6 months. The design is puzzling. Why would something you are not consuming lower your risk for depression? Then authors also noted that Japanese women already have high fish intake.

A study from Singapore recruited 698 mothers at 26 to 28 weeks' gestation and measured their plasma levels of omega-3s and 6s (Chong et al., 2015). They measured depression and anxiety in pregnancy and at 3 months postpartum. The overall rate of depression was only 7% during pregnancy, with a very high EPDS cutoff (>15), and 10% postpartum with a high cutoff (>13). Low omega-3s and a higher omega-6 to omega-3 ratio were associated with higher anxiety during pregnancy, but not postpartum, and with depression in pregnancy or postpartum. Low omega-3s were related to high levels of inflammation. Their findings are consistent with previous studies examining the link between inflammation and anxiety.

Treatment with EPA and DHA

A recent review of 18 randomized clinical trials (N = 4,052) found that there was an overall positive effect of omega-3s on depressive symptoms in perinatal women (Mocking et al., 2020). However, there was substantial heterogeneity in findings. If women were depressed, omega-3s had a medium effect but had no effect for non-depressed women. In addition, omega-3s had a medium to large effect in postpartum women but a negligible effect during pregnancy. The studies of postpartum depression showed the strongest effect. The authors recommended omega-3s as a promising add-on treatment. They concluded that EPA is more effective than DHA as a treatment for postpartum depression. DHA could be useful during pregnancy for other things, such as preterm birth, child allergy, or child neurodevelopment. However, DHA does not treat depression. Both this study and an older review of 10 articles (Wojcicki & Heyman, 2011) concluded that higher doses were more effective.

A report by the American Psychiatric Association's Omega-3 Fatty Acids Subcommittee found a protective effect of EPA and DHA on mood disorders (Freeman et al., 2006a). They also noted that omega-3 supplementation could counter some of the metabolic and obesity effects of medications for psychiatric conditions.

A review article from Italy included 36 RCTs on omega-3 supplementation on unipolar and bipolar depression and depression during pregnancy (Ciappolino et al., 2017). EPA was more effective in treating depression than DHA. They concluded that "some evidence" supported the efficacy of EPA in affective disorders but that the studies were not powered enough to confirm a therapeutic effect. Interestingly, they found that omega-3s helped with bipolar disorder, but not perinatal depression. In examining their results more closely, they based their findings on perinatal depression from 7 studies, 4 of which either focused entirely on DHA or the EPA levels were below the therapeutic dose. Of the remaining 3 studies, 1 had significant findings and the other 2 did not. However, the sample size for the three studies ranged from 26 to 59, which could have also limited the power of the studies to detect a difference.

A review from Australia found that EPA effectively treated depression in 4 of the 6 studies reviewed. One gram of EPA per day was the effective dose. Doses higher than 2 grams were too much and seemed to increase depression. Their findings suggest an optimum dose, and exceeding it makes it less effective (Rees et al., 2005). Similarly, in a meta-analysis of 10 studies ($N = 329$), EPA with DHA had a significant antidepressant effect for patients with depression and with bipolar disorder (Lin & Su, 2007). However, Lin and Su noted methodologic limitations in the studies they cited.

EPA and DHA were also used to treat major depression during pregnancy (Su et al., 2008). This randomized trial of 36 pregnant women with major depression compared a placebo to 3.4 grams EPA/DHA (2.2 grams DHA, 1.2 grams EPA). Women in the EPA/DHA group had significantly lower depression scores on the Hamilton Depression Rating Scale at 6 and 8 weeks than those in the placebo group. Their remission rate was also higher, but this difference was not significant. Mothers tolerated EPA and DHA well, and there were no adverse effects for either mother or baby. EPA and DHA may have halted the arachidonic acid cascade, which is often higher in the plasma of people with depression and is a proinflammatory omega-6 fatty acid.

Hallahan and colleagues (2007) tested whether EPA/DHA helped patients who had attempted suicide more than once. Participants were recruited from London emergency departments. Forty-nine patients received either a placebo or 1.2 grams EPA and 900 milligrams DHA. After 12 weeks, the EPA/DHA patients were less depressed and had lower daily stresses. EPA/DHA also lowered suicide risk, as indicated by significant markers for suicidality.

Effective Dosage of EPA

According to the previously cited reviews, EPA is the only omega-3 that treats depression. DHA can be added to EPA, but it should never be used as a monotreatment for depression. The next question pertains to dosage. Several studies have recommended a specific dosage of EPA, which ranges between 1 and 2 grams. For example, Wojcicki and Heyman (2011) recommended 2 grams of EPA and DHA, while Mocking and colleagues (2020) recommended 2.2 grams of EPA only.

EPA was used for depressive symptoms in bipolar disorder in a 12-week double-blind trial (Frangou et al., 2006). Seventy-five patients were randomly assigned to either placebo, 1 gram, or 2 grams of EPA. After 12 weeks, both EPA groups improved substantially compared to the placebo. One gram was as effective as 2, and there was no advantage to 2 grams over 1 gram. Similarly, an Australian review compared 1 vs. 2 grams of EPA and found that 1 gram was as effective as 2 (Rees et al., 2005). They felt that the extra EPA in 2 grams might become counterproductive.

At this point, it is difficult to say whether 1 gram is the optimal dose or if more is needed. Clinicians may opt to start with 1 gram of EPA and assess within a month. Another gram could be safely added. Effective dose will be influenced by patient weight, age, sex, and other medications they are taking.

Why They Work: Stress, Inflammation, and EPA

EPA lowers proinflammatory cytokines, and this likely explains its efficacy in treating depression. It also moderates the inflammatory action of arachidonic acid by competing for the same metabolic pathways (Chong et al., 2015; Ciappolino et al., 2017; Noorbakhshnia et al., 2015 {Chong, 2015 #2855}). In a large population study, high levels of omega-3s (ALA, EPA, and DHA) in participants' plasma were related to lower levels of the proinflammatory cytokines IL-1α, IL-1β, IL-6, and TNF-α and higher levels of anti-inflammatory cytokines, such as IL-10. For people with low levels of omega-3s, the opposite was true: these people had high levels of proinflammatory cytokines and low levels of anti-inflammatory cytokines (Ferrucci et al., 2006).

EPA and DHA also impact the stress system. Maes and colleagues (2000) found that college students with deficient levels of EPA/DHA had a stronger inflammatory response when exposed to a lab-induced stressor compared to non-deficient students and were more resilient. Kiecolt-Glaser and colleagues (2007) found that a history of depression or trauma "primes" the inflammatory response system in their study of 43 older adults, which made them more vulnerable to subsequent stress (Kiecolt-Glaser et al., 2015). However, even modest levels of supplementation with EPA and DHA lowered norepinephrine.

In a study from Japan, participants took either a placebo or 762 milligrams of EPA/DHA for 2 months in this double-blind trial (Hamazaki et al., 2005). The researchers noted that EPA concentrations increased in the red blood cell membranes in the supplemented group. The EPA/DHA group also had significantly decreased levels of plasma norepinephrine.

In another Japanese study, 83 participants 10 days after they had a car accident were given either a placebo or 1,470 milligrams of DHA/147 milligrams of EPA (Matsumura et al., 2017). They continued for 12 weeks. The researchers hypothesized that omega-3s extinguished fear memories by facilitating hippocampal neurogenesis via the endocannabinoid system, and that they reduced sympathetic nervous system activity. Heart rate was the outcome variable, at rest and under stress. There were no differences between the groups at baseline. At 12 weeks, the omega-3 group had a significantly lower heart rate than those in the placebo group. The authors proposed omega-3s may prevent some of the psychophysiological symptoms of PTSD.

In summary, EPA and DHA downregulate the stress response, and by doing so, these fatty acids help mothers become more resilient to stress. This is especially valuable for women who are highly stressed or who have experienced trauma, as EPA and DHA increase resilience to stress and can decrease risk for postpartum depression (Kendall-Tackett, 2007).

DHA in the Perinatal Period

DHA does not treat depression, but it may help prevent it. It is particularly important during pregnancy. In many Western countries, pregnant women's diets are deficient in DHA. This is a problem because babies need high amounts of DHA in the last trimester of pregnancy for their brain and vision development. Any stores of DHA that mothers have are diverted to their babies, which increases mothers' risk for depression. As Rees and colleagues (2005) describe for mothers in Australia, during the last trimester of pregnancy, babies accumulate an average of 67 milligrams per day of DHA. The average intake for Australian mothers is 15 milligrams per day. In contrast, DHA consumption from diet is about 1,000 milligrams per day for Japanese, Koreans, and Norwegians, all countries with high fish consumption.

A double-blind, randomized trial with 2,399 pregnant women in Australia found that DHA supplementation did not prevent postpartum depression, nor did it improve child cognitive or language development at 12 to 18 months (Makrides et al., 2010). The negative results may be due to the study design. Women were recruited at 21 weeks' gestation. They received either 800 milligrams DHA and 100 milligrams EPA or a vegetable oil placebo until birth, and then they stopped taking it. Why would something mothers are *not taking* lower their risk for depression? And there are many things that contribute to children's cognitive development. It is not as simple as taking a pill. DHA, however, did do something really important: it increased gestation length.

The current recommended minimum dose is 200 to 400 milligrams per day. This may prove to be too low a dose to prevent depression. According to McNamara (2009), in order to prevent affective disorders, you need a 7% erythrocyte DHA level, which can be achieved with an adult dose of 700 to 1,000 milligrams. Interestingly, that amount is similar to the amount of DHA that women who eat a lot of fish consume through diet in countries, such as Japan or Norway (Rees et al., 2005).

DHA Lowers the Risk for Preterm Birth

As I described in Volume I, depression, anxiety, and PTSD during pregnancy increase risk for preterm birth, the second leading cause of infant mortality worldwide (Centers for Disease Control, 2019). Anecdotally, I learned that the rate of preterm birth was markedly increased during COVID-19. I suspect the rise is due to the same mechanism: the stress-related increase in inflammation.

Inflammation underlies depression, anxiety, chronic stress, and PTSD and is the physiological mechanism that increases the risk of preterm birth. As one recent review states, "human studies have implicated IL-1, TNF, and IL-6 as major players in PTB [preterm birth]" (Cappelletti et al., 2016). Cousson-Read and colleagues' (2012) study of 173 women found that those who had preterm babies had higher IL-6 and TNF-α compared with women who delivered at term. The rate of preterm birth was 11%. The researchers noted that prenatal stress increases the number of proinflammatory cytokines, which shortens gestation. IL-6 and TNF-α also ripen the cervix (Coussons-Read et al., 2005).

Fortunately, DHA, because of its anti-inflammatory action, blocks the action of IL-6 and TNF-α and increases gestation length (Makrides et al., 2010; Smuts, 2003). The most convincing evidence if from a Cochrane Review of 70 RCTs (N = 19,927) on omega-3 supplementation during pregnancy. The review concluded that "omega-3 supplementation during pregnancy is an effective strategy for reducing the incidence of preterm birth" (Middleton et al., 2018). The evidence was so compelling that they further concluded that more studies are not needed at this stage.

Safety During Pregnancy and Lactation

EPA and DHA supplements are generally safe for peripartum women (Makrides et al., 2010; Marangell et al., 2004; Shoji et al., 2006). A few studies have found very mild negative effects at high-dose levels, but in most studies, there are no adverse effects. These findings are summarized in the following sections.

Pregnancy Studies

Many studies on EPA and DHA are based on population studies examining fish consumption. One study sampled 182 women from the Faroe Islands: a whaling island community between the Shetland Islands and Iceland (Grandjean et al., 2001). Among Faroe Islanders, fish consumption was high: 72 grams of fish, 12 grams of whale muscle, and 7 grams of whale blubber per day. In this sample, DHA level was the best predictor of gestational length, with a 1% increase in relative concentration related to a 1.5-day increase in gestation. An increase of 1% in relative EPA concentration was related to a 246-gram decrease in birthweight. This decrease was not clinically significant, however, given the generally high birthweights of babies born in the Faroe Islands.

A study of 488 women in Iceland found that women who took cod-liver oil were at increased risk for developing hypertension in pregnancy (Olafsdottir et al., 2006). That finding, as presented in the article abstract, is somewhat misleading. In the full article, the authors noted that when the data were divided into centiles, a U-shaped curve showed that women at the highest and lowest levels of supplementation were most at risk for hypertension. Women with modest levels of supplementation had the lowest risk, suggesting a possible optimal dose. Too much or too little increased risk. In addition, cod-liver oil also contains vitamins A, D, and E, which can be toxic if too much is taken, so large doses would be a problem. Finally, cod-liver oil consumption was measured via questionnaire, not from participant serum.

Modest levels of cod-liver oil supplementation appeared safe in another randomized trial of 341 women, where mothers were supplemented from 18 weeks' gestation to 3 months postpartum (803 milligrams EPA, 1,183 milligrams DHA) (Helland, 2003). No teratogenic effects were noted. All babies breastfed for at least 3 months. At age 4, children whose mothers took cod-liver oil during pregnancy and lactation had a higher Mental Processing Composite score.

Another study examined whether fish consumption during pregnancy protected offspring from allergic disease (Romieu et al., 2007). The rationale was that omega-3s were anti-inflammatory, which moderates the immune system. The sample included 462 pregnant women and their infants who were followed until age 6. After adjusting for confounding variables, they found that fish intake during pregnancy protected infants from eczema at 1 year, and allergy and wheeze at 6 years. An increase in weekly fish from once to 2.5 times a week decreased the risk of eczema by 37%, and risk of positive skin prick test at age 6 by 35%. Risk was significantly lowered for non-breastfed children. For breastfeeding mothers, fish consumption provided no added benefit.

In a meta-analysis, Szajewska et al. (2006) found that the incidence of adverse effects from EPA/DHA supplementation was low. Most adverse effects were mild (e.g., fish burps). One study included in the review reported an increase in blood loss at delivery among the fish-oil group, but none of the other studies found this. Across studies, they found no difference in adverse effects between supplemented and non-supplemented neonates.

Breastfeeding Studies

EPA and DHA also appear to have no negative impact on breastfeeding babies, even at high dosages. Freeman and colleagues (2006b) conducted a small randomized trial using three different dosages of EPA/DHA with 16 mothers with postpartum major depression

(300 milligrams EPA/200 milligrams DHA, 840 milligrams EPA/560 milligrams DHA, or 1,680 milligrams EPA/1,120 milligrams DHA). Depression significantly decreased in all three groups, and there were no adverse effects noted for mother or baby at any dosage level.

In a sample of 83 mothers, EPA and DHA made small changes in breastmilk fatty acid composition when mothers were supplemented from 20 weeks' gestation to delivery. These changes appeared to be beneficial, however, not harmful. Fish-oil supplementation significantly increased EPA and DHA concentrations in breastmilk (Dunstan, Roper, et al., 2004), and in the erythrocytes of mothers and babies in the fish-oil group (Dunstan, Mori, et al., 2004). High EPA/DHA increased IgA and sCD14 in the milk, potentially protective changes. The dose used in this study was high (2.2 grams DHA, 1.5 grams EPA): *11 times* the recommended minimum of DHA. Dunstan and colleagues expressed some concerns about what the alterations in fatty acid composition might mean, but their concerns were more hypothetical than observed.

Sources of EPA and DHA

How can women safely increase their EPA and DHA levels while pregnant or breastfeeding? Fish is a key source (and possibly, the only source of EPA). Yet fish might be contaminated by pollution, which could harm their developing infants. Although I generally think that food is the best way to get nutrients, in this case, fish-oil supplements are safer, especially during pregnancy. In the United States, the US Pharmacopeia tests brands of fish-oil products and verifies ones that are safe. There are likely similar non-industry organizations in other countries that test local brands. If safe brands are not available locally, mothers can likely find them online. There are also vegetarian DHA products that are not contaminated. (The US Pharmacopeia website lists specific brands that are tested for contaminants and are USP-verified: www.USP.org.)

Summary

Evidence is mixed in terms of using EPA as a monotherapy, but it has an important role as an adjunct to other therapies. DHA should not be used as a monotherapy, but it helps prevent depression and lowers the risk of preterm birth. There are many health benefits from correcting deficiencies of EPA and DHA, with no apparent harm. A review in the *British Journal of Psychiatry* summarized these findings as follows:

> There is good evidence that psychiatric illness is associated with the depletion of EFAs [essential fatty acids] and, crucially, that supplementation can result in clinical amelioration. . . . The clinical trial data may herald a simple, safe and effective adjunct to our standard treatments.
>
> (Hallahan & Garland, 2005, p. 276)

Clinical Takeaways

- I recommend all mothers supplement with omega-3s because they have many health benefits, with few documented harms (possible blood thinning was cited, but this has not be documented). Both EPA and DHA lower proinflammatory cytokines.

- Supplementing with DHA during pregnancy can lower risk for preterm birth.
- EPA is the omega-3 that treats depression.
- DHA does not treat but can be a useful adjunct. The recommended dose of 200 milligrams is likely too low. Mothers in countries with high fish consumption generally get 800 to 1,000 milligrams through their diets. This may prove to be a more efficacious dose.
- Fish oil is the only source of EPA (so far), but vegetarian forms of DHA are available.

9 Nutraceuticals II

Vitamin D, Vitamin B-12, Curcumin, and St. John's Wort

Four additional nutraceuticals have shown promise in preventing and treating perinatal depression. With vitamins D and B-12, testing mothers and supplementing them if they are deficient improves their physical and mental health. Curcumin, the principal ingredient in turmeric, shows promise for treating inflammatory diseases, including depression. St. John's wort is a botanical antidepressant and is highly anti-inflammatory. If used with care, it has an excellent safety record.

KEY FINDINGS

- Many mothers are vitamin D deficient. Deficiency increases inflammation, which increases their risk for depression.
- Similarly, mothers with B-12 deficiencies have a higher risk for depression. Vegans and women who have had gastric bypass surgery are more at higher risk for B-12 deficiencies.
- Curcumin shows promise as a treatment for depression in the general population. However, research is limited with perinatal women.
- St. John's wort is a botanical antidepressant that has a good side effect profile and is safe for breastfeeding. However, it should not be mixed with other prescription medications, particularly antidepressants.

Vitamin D

Vitamin D is a preprohormone that influences metabolism and immune function. Pregnant and postpartum women worldwide are vitamin D deficient. This deficiency is partly because we spend so much time indoors and partly because our reasonable efforts to prevent skin cancer block our access to *any* sun.

When people are deficient in vitamin D, they are more vulnerable to inflammatory diseases, such as rheumatoid arthritis, cardiovascular disease, and diabetes (Wagner et al., 2010). Vitamin D protects beta cell function from inflammatory cytokines, particularly IL-6 and TNF-α (Penckofer et al., 2008). When it is deficient, IL-6 inhibits insulin receptor signal transduction. IL-6 is associated with hyperglycemia and hyperinsulinemia. Given that a deficiency in vitamin D increases inflammation, it is not surprising that it has a role in depression (Berk et al., 2013). A recent review of meta-analysis on complementary treatments for depression found that vitamin D was an effective treatment for depression, but the quality of evidence was low (Haller et al., 2019). Vitamin D deficiency also reduces intestinal calcium absorption by more than 50%, causing the

DOI: 10.4324/9781003405092-11

parathyroid to correct the calcium imbalance by releasing calcium from the bones. Hyperparathyroidism is another way that vitamin D deficiency increases risk for cardio-vascular disease (Academy of Breastfeeding Medicine, 2008).

Vitamin D is measured via serum: 25-hydroxyvitamin D (ng/ml). Severe deficiency is <10, deficient = 10–20, insufficient = 21–29, and sufficient = >30. Toxic levels are >150 (Academy of Breastfeeding Medicine, 2008). Standard recommended supplements are 400 IU per day for adults. However, newer guidelines are emerging, with the recommended dosage for pregnant women being 4,000 IU/day, and 6,400 IU for lactating women (Wagner, 2011). These recommendations follow from Wagner et al.'s earlier clinical trials demonstrating that these high levels are safe, and not toxic, for pregnant and postpartum women (Wagner et al., 2006).

Vitamin D and Postpartum Depression

A recent study of 1,773 participants from urban China included 907 breastfeeding women and 866 pregnant women (Wang et al., 2023). The overall prevalence of prenatal depression was 16%, and postpartum depression was 10%. Twenty-seven percent had vitamin D deficiency. Wang et al. compared women who were vitamin D deficient to non-deficient women. The postpartum women who were vitamin D deficient were 70% more likely to have depressive symptoms. Their serum vitamin D levels were inversely related their scores on the Edinburgh Postnatal Depression Scale. (The lower the vitamin D levels, the higher their score.) Sleep quality was also negatively correlated with vitamin D deficiency, which was indirectly related to depression. Interestingly, they speculated that the Chinese practice of confining women to bed for several weeks, where they do not go out, could contribute to the vitamin D deficiency. There was not a similar finding for pregnant women.

A prospective study of 796 pregnant women from Perth, Australia (a very sunny place), measured vitamin D levels at 18 weeks' gestation, and measured depression at 3 days postpartum (Robinson et al., 2014). The researchers used 6 items from the EPDS that measured mood fluctuations, sadness, anxiety, appetite changes, and sleep disturbances. As hypothesized, women in the lowest quartile for vitamin D had the most depressive symptoms, even after accounting for potentially confounding variables, such as BMI and demographic factors.

A systematic review examined 7 studies that assessed the relationship between vitamin D and postpartum depression (Amini et al., 2019). Vitamin D deficiency was related to incidence of postpartum depression and was significant in recovery. They noted that none of the studies were randomized trials. They were all observational studies that compared postpartum depression and existing vitamin D status, without giving women vitamin D as an intervention. Six were prospective cohort studies, and one was cross-sectional.

Although finds are mixed with regard to depression, there is no downside to correcting a vitamin D deficiency.

Vitamin B-12

Vitamin B-12 deficiency also increases the risk of inflammatory conditions. Deficiencies in pyridoxine (B-6) and cobalamin (B-12) are associated with increased homocysteine, a proinflammatory amino acid. A recent study from India examined 217 women with possible postpartum depression and compared them with 217 non-depressed women who were matched for age and BMI (Dhiman et al., 2021). If B-12 is low, 5-HT (serotonin) becomes less bioavailable and homocysteine accumulates, which can lead to depression. They found that B-12 levels were significantly lower in women with postpartum depression and methylmalonic acid and 5-methyl THF were significantly higher than for women in the comparison group. Women with the lowest B-12 levels were 4.53 times more likely to be depressed.

Curcumin

Curcumin is the principal curcuminoid in the spice turmeric and is highly anti-inflammatory. Curcumin blocks the formation of reactive oxygen species and inhibits cyclooxygenase 1 and 2 (COX-1 and -2) (Peng et al., 2021). (Medications, such as ibuprofen, also inhibit COX enzymes.) Curcumin influences the HPA axis, the inflammatory response system, and nitrosative and oxidative stress (Lopresti et al., 2014). It specifically decreases levels of the proinflammatory cytokines related to depression (IL-1β, IL-6, and TNF-α) and C-reactive protein. It also results in increased excretion of proinflammatory arachidonic acid and substance P, the neuropeptide associated with pain (Peng et al., 2021).

Because it downregulated the stress and inflammatory response systems, curcumin was hypothesized as a possible treatment for major depressive disorder. Its anti-inflammatory properties are considered the basis for its role in treating disease. It has been studied as a treatment of inflammatory diseases such as arthritis and for depression, atherosclerosis, and COVID-19.

In a double-blind, placebo-controlled study, 56 non-postpartum adults with major depressive disorder were randomized to treatment with 500 milligrams of curcumin twice daily or a placebo (Lopresti et al., 2014). At 4 weeks, people in both conditions improved, but from 4 to 8 weeks, curcumin was significantly more effective at alleviating depression than the placebo. Curcumin significantly lowered total depressive symptoms, arousal-related symptoms, and trait anxiety. It did not significantly differ from the placebo before 4 weeks. The effects were strongest for people with atypical depression. Atypical depression is characterized by higher levels of inflammation (C-reactive protein, IL-6, and TNF-α). Curcumin lowers CRP, IL-6, and TNFα.

A recent meta-analysis of curcumin and depression found that it significantly lowered depressive (10 studies, $N = 531$) and anxiety (5 studies, $N = 284$) symptoms (Fusar-Poli et al., 2020). There was a large effect size, and it was generally well tolerated. The authors suggested adding it to standard care might improve symptoms in people with depression.

Curcumin reduced the effects of prenatal exposure to endocrine disruptors, such as bisphenol A (BPA). In animal studies, curcumin ameliorated diabetes in pregnant mice. However, the authors expressed some concern about the safety of its use during pregnancy without more complete data (Filardi et al., 2020).

Some mothers use curcumin as a galactagogue (a substance that increases milk production), but caution is warranted. An in vitro study of lactating mammary epithelial cells found that curcumin downregulated milk production in these cells by inactivating the STAT5 and GR signaling with concurrent suppression of inflammatory responses (Kobayashi et al., 2021). On the other hand, a topical curcumin cream significantly reduced breast inflammation in a randomized double-blind, placebo-controlled study from Oman (Afshariani et al., 2014). After 72 hours, mothers in the curcumin group had significantly lower rates of moderate or mild mastitis, with significantly lower scores for breast tension, erythema, and pain.

St. John's Wort

St. John's wort (*Hypericum perforatum)* is the most widely used herbal antidepressant in the world (Dugoua et al., 2006). It contains hypericin, hyperforin, and flavonoids, such as quercetin (LactMed, 2021). Herbalists have used St. John's wort since the Middle Ages, when it was used to treat insanity resulting from "attacks of the devil." It derives its name from St. John's Day (June 24) because it blooms near this day on the medieval church calendar. "Wort" is the old English word for a medicinal plant. It is native to Great Britain, Wales, and northern Europe. Since settlers brought it to North America in the 1700s, it is now a common wildflower in the Northeastern and North Central United States.

Efficacy of St. John's Wort

Several clinical trials compared the efficacy of St. John's wort to either placebos or antidepressants. In one trial, 375 patients were randomized to receive either St. John's wort (*Hypericum perforatum* extract WS 5570) or a placebo for 6 weeks to treat mild to moderate depression (Lecrubier et al., 2002). At the end of 6 weeks, patients receiving St. John's wort had significantly lower scores on the Hamilton Depression Rating Scale. Significantly more patients were in remission than those receiving the placebo. Both groups had similar rates of adverse effects. Fifty-three percent of the patients in the St. John's wort group responded to treatment, compared with 42% of the placebo group (a high percentage for a placebo effect).

Another randomized trial compared St. John's wort (*Hypericum* extract ZE 117) to the tricyclic antidepressant imipramine for 324 outpatients with mild to moderate depression (Woelk, 2000). After 6 weeks of treatment, St. John's wort was as effective as imipramine in lowering depressive symptoms. Adverse effects were significantly higher in the imipramine group, with 63% reporting adverse effects compared with 39% reporting adverse effects in the St. John's wort group. In addition, only 3% in the St. John's wort group dropped out of the study due to adverse effects vs. 16% of the imipramine group. The author concluded that St. John's wort is therapeutically equivalent to imipramine but better tolerated by patients.

Two clinical trials compared St. John's wort to sertraline for major depression. In the first study, 340 adults with major depression were randomly assigned to receive *H. perforatum*, a placebo, or sertraline for 8 weeks (Hypericum Depression Trial Study Group, 2002). Subjects responding to the medication could opt to receive still-blinded treatment for another 18 weeks. Depression was assessed at baseline, and again at 8 weeks. The rate of full response was low and almost identical for both the St. John's wort and sertraline groups (24% vs. 25%). The low response rates for both medications suggest limitations to the study. Eight weeks may not have been sufficient for patients with severe depression to recover. Or the dosages may have been too low. The authors noted that their findings were not unusual in that approximately 35% of studies of standard antidepressants show no greater efficacy than the placebo. (It is important to understand that antidepressants do not work for everyone. Monitoring is important to ensure that treatments work.)

Another study had different findings (Van Gurp et al., 2002). This study included 87 patients with major depression recruited from Canadian family practice physicians. Patients were randomly assigned to receive either St. John's wort or sertraline. At the end of the 12-week trial, both groups improved, and there was no difference between the two groups. However, the sertraline group had significantly more side effects at 2 and 4 weeks. The authors concluded that St. John's wort, because of its effectiveness and benign side effects, was a good *first choice* for a primary care population.

St. John's wort was also compared to paroxetine in a study of 251 patients with moderate to severe major depression (Szegedi et al., 2005). In this study, patients were randomly assigned to receive 20 milligrams paroxetine or 900 milligrams St. John's wort (*Hypericum* extract WS 5570). After 2 weeks, dosages for non-responders were doubled: 1,800 milligrams St. John's wort or 40 milligrams paroxetine. After 6 weeks of treatment, the response rates were 70% for St. John's wort and 60% for paroxetine. The remission rates for St. John's wort were 50% vs. 35% for paroxetine. The authors concluded that St. John's wort was as effective as paroxetine and better tolerated.

Anghelescu and colleagues (2006) also compared the efficacy and safety of *Hypericum* extract WS 5570 to paroxetine for patients with moderate to severe depression. The acute phase of treatment lasted for 6 weeks, with another 4 months of follow-up to prevent relapse. The patients improved on both treatments, with no significant difference in efficacy between paroxetine and St. John's wort. The authors noted that St. John's wort was an important alternative to standard antidepressants.

A recent meta-analysis of 26 meta-analyses of randomized trials found a moderate quality of evidence supporting the efficacy of St. John's wort vs. a placebo for treating mild to major depression (Haller et al., 2019). St. John's wort caused significantly fewer adverse effects than antidepressants. In contrast, medications and psychotherapy, the traditional treatment recommendation for depression, had high dropout rates and low remission rates.

Mechanism for Efficacy

Researchers still do not understand why St. John's wort works. They recognized hyperforin as the possible antidepressant constituent (Lawvere & Mahoney, 2005; Wurglies & Schubert-Zsilavecz, 2006). Hyperforin appears to inhibit the reuptake of the monoamine neurotransmitters and GABAergic activity (Deligiannidis & Freeman, 2014). St. John's wort may relieve depression by preventing the reuptake of serotonin, the same mechanism as the selective-serotonin reuptake inhibitors (SSRIs) (e.g., fluoxetine, sertraline). Indeed, only hyperforin (and its structural analogue, adhyperforin) inhibits neurotransmitter reuptake (Muller, 2003).

St. John's wort, and particularly hyperforin, lowers inflammation (Dell'Aica et al., 2007; Wurglies & Schubert-Zsilavecz, 2006), and it modulates cytokine production (Werneke et al., 2006). Hyperforin has had anti-nociceptive (anti-pain) and anti-inflammatory effects in animal studies (Abdel-Salam, 2005). It inhibits the expression of another inflammatory marker—intercellular adhesion molecule (Zhou et al., 2004). In vitro effects show that St. John's wort is antioxidant, anti-cyclooxygenase-1, and anti-carcinogenic (Zanoli, 2004). The study used an animal model to test whether St. John's wort could counter the toxic side effects of chemotherapy. The investigators specifically investigated whether St. John's wort had an impact on the levels of proinflammatory cytokines, including IL-1β, IL-2, IL-6, IFN-γ, and TNF-α. They found that St. John's wort did inhibit proinflammatory cytokines and intestinal epithelium apoptosis. Although not a study of depression, it was the first to demonstrate that St. John's wort inhibits the cytokines that are high in depression (Hu et al., 2006).

Dosage

The dosage of St. John's wort is 900 milligrams per day (300 milligrams, three times per day), standardized to 0.3% hypericin and/or 2% to 4% hyperforin (Lawvere & Mahoney, 2005). It generally takes 4 to 6 weeks to take effect (Ernst, 2002). St. John's wort reaches peak level in the plasma in 5 hours, with a half-life of 24 to 48 hours. Herbalists often combine it with other herbs to address the range of symptoms that depressed people have. Some of these herbs include lemon balm, kava, schisandra, rosemary, black cohosh, and lavender (Humphrey, 2007; Kuhn & Winston, 2000).

Unfortunately, in the United States, it can be challenging for women to know if herbs they purchase are good quality. The US Pharmacopeia sells a powdered St. John's wort, but it is expensive. ConsumerLabs.com rates brands of herbs. In countries like Germany, where St. John's wort is regulated and is part of their healthcare system, it is an excellent option. However, in countries where there is no oversight, I am concerned that consumers may purchase an ineffective or harmful product. More concerning, they may not tell their healthcare provider that they are taking it, which can lead to serious consequences.

Safety Concerns

Taken by itself, St. John's wort has an excellent safety record, with a very low frequency of adverse reactions (Humphrey, 2007; Muller, 2003). Approximately 2% of patients who take St. John's wort develop side effects. The most common are mild stomach discomfort, allergic reactions, skin rashes, tiredness, and restlessness. Like other antidepressants, St. John's wort can trigger an episode of mania in patients with underlying bipolar disorder (Bratman & Girman, 2003). St. John's wort can also cause photosensitivity. A review of 38 controlled clinical trials and two meta-analyses on St. John's wort found its safety and side effect profile to be better than those of standard antidepressants. The incidence of adverse events ranged from 0% to 6% (Schultz, 2006). There is also a significantly lower dropout rate in studies due to side effects in SJW trials vs. studies of antidepressants.

A safety concern is that St. John's wort interacts with several classes of medications. Studies suggest that the mechanism likely involves the drug-metabolizing enzyme CYP3A4 and the transport protein P-glycoprotein (Schultz, 2006). This enzyme accelerates the metabolism of anticoagulants, anticonvulsants, cyclosporins, birth control pills, protease and reverse transcriptase inhibitors used in anti-HIV treatments, and others, leading to lower serum levels of the medication than prescribed (Ernst, 2002; Schultz, 2006). It can also interact with prescription antidepressants, causing a potentially fatal episode of serotonin syndrome (Looper, 2007; Schultz, 2006). Prescription antidepressants should not be taken while taking St. John's wort (Harkness & Bratman, 2003). Mothers who are taking St. John's wort need to tell their healthcare providers to ensure that it is safe.

St. John's Wort and Breastfeeding

St. John's wort is generally safe to take while breastfeeding (Dugoua et al., 2006; Hale, 2021; LactMed, 2021) and is generally below the limit of detection in infants whose mothers took SJW up to 22 weeks (LactMed, 2021). Infants whose mothers used St. John's wort had normal assessment scores, and it did not seem to influence either prolactin and/or milk production. The average dosage from 36 hind- and foremilk samples was 1.5%.

In a case study, Klier and colleagues (2002) examined the pharmacokinetics of St. John's wort in four breastmilk samples from a mother taking the standard dose (300 milligrams, three times per day). They tested the samples for both hypericin and hyperforin and found that only hyperforin was excreted into breastmilk at a low level. Both hyperforin and hypericin were below the level of quantification in the infant's plasma.

Klier and colleagues (2006) tested 36 breastmilk samples from five mothers taking 300 milligrams of St. John's wort, three times a day. They also tested the plasma of the five mothers and two infants. As with their earlier case study, they found that only hyperforin was excreted into breastmilk, at low levels. The relative infant dose of hyperforin was 1% to 3% of the mother's dose, a level of infant exposure comparable to antidepressants. No side effects were noted in either mothers or babies.

There is good evidence to support use of St. John's wort while breastfeeding (Dugoua et al., 2006). The authors found that St. John's wort affects neither milk supply nor infant weight. They noted that it could cause infant colic, drowsiness, or lethargy, although only a few cases have been reported. They concluded that common and traditional use of St. John's wort caused minimal risk for breastfeeding women and their babies. They did express some concern about use of St. John's wort during pregnancy, however. Given the other choices for treatment, avoiding it while pregnant is prudent.

Summary

Findings on vitamins D and B-12 suggest screening as many women around the world are deficient. Vitamin D and/or B-12 deficiency increases susceptibility to a wide range of chronic health conditions because they increase inflammation. Deficiency has also been linked to perinatal depression. Addressing vitamin D and B-12 deficiency can prevent depression or help women heal once it has occurred.

Curcumin is an emerging treatment with promising results in non-postpartum adults. It, too, is anti-inflammatory and has efficacy for many physical health conditions. Not as much is known about its effects on pregnancy and lactation. So far, no negative effects have been identified. Some worry that it may act as a blood thinner, but that is more of a theoretical vs. actual risk. It is one to watch because using it to treat depression helps physical health as well.

Finally, St. John's wort is another effective treatment for depression. Its standard use is for mild to moderate depression, but studies have also used it for major depression. However, some cautions are in order. Even though St. John's wort is a "natural" alternative to medications, it *is* a medication and should be treated as such. **It should never be used with commercial antidepressants.**

In addition, mothers should tell their healthcare providers that they are taking it, as it can interact with several different medications. If used with safety concerns in mind, normal use does not appear to be harmful for mothers or babies, but some caution has been raised about use during pregnancy, so it seems prudent to avoid. Although hyperforin is excreted into breastmilk, it appears in very low levels in infant plasma and in some cases was undetectable (Hale, 2021).

Clinical Takeaways

- Testing mothers for vitamins B-12 and D deficiency improves mothers' physical health by lowering inflammation, which lowers their risk for depression. I recommend testing all mothers who screen positive for depression. You might also want to order a complete blood test to rule out anemia, especially if a mother hemorrhaged after her delivery.

- Curcumin supports physical health and lowers the risk for many inflammation-based disorders. It is also a promising treatment for depression.
- St. John's wort is a safe and effective alternative to antidepressants. However, it may be difficult to get quality products in countries where herbal products are not regulated, such as the United States. Women should tell their healthcare providers that they are taking St. John's wort, especially if they are taking other medications. St. John's wort may be "natural," but it is a medication and should be treated accordingly.

10 Exercise

Exercise is bit like flossing; people know they "should" do it but often do not. However, for treating depression, exercise is a great option (Daley et al., 2007). Traditionally, practitioners recommend exercise for milder depressions but feel that they must bring out the "big guns" (i.e., medications) for anything more serious. Many clinicians would be surprised to learn that exercise went head-to-head with medications in randomized trials and was as effective—even for major depression. In addition, exercise can also be safely combined with other modalities and is likely more acceptable as a treatment option (Reza et al., 2018). The mood-altering effects of exercise appear quickly. In a study of 26 women, Lane and colleagues (2002) found that women's moods significantly improved after each exercise session. Depressed mood was especially sensitive to exercise and decreased significantly after each session.

KEY FINDINGS

- Exercise treats even major depression and is as effective as sertraline in reducing symptoms. Patients in the exercise group were also less likely to relapse.
- Exercise during pregnancy and postpartum lowers mothers' risk for depression and reduces depressive symptoms.
- Regular exercise lowers inflammation.

Exercise as a Treatment for Depression

Researchers at the Duke University Medical Center were the first to pit exercise against sertraline for major depression (Babyak et al., 2000; Blumenthal et al., 2007). In the first study, 156 adults with major depression (>50 years old) were randomized into one of three treatment groups: aerobic exercise alone, sertraline alone, and a combination of exercise and sertraline. After 4 months, exercise was as effective as sertraline in alleviating depression. The more striking findings, however, occurred at 10 months. People in the exercise-only group had a significantly lower rate of relapse than those in the medication-only or the medication/exercise groups. The authors speculated that participants in the exercise-only group had learned that exercise was a coping tool that they could use when facing life stressors. The exercise/medication group may have attributed their recovery more to medication than exercise.

These same researchers replicated their findings with a larger sample (Blumenthal et al., 2007). Two-hundred twenty adults with major depression were randomized to one of four conditions: sertraline, exercise at home, supervised exercise, or a placebo

DOI: 10.4324/9781003405092-12

control. After 4 months of treatment, 41% of the patients were in remission and no longer met the criteria for major depression. Efficacy rates by treatment were as follows: medication = 47%, supervised exercise = 45%, home-based exercise = 40%, and placebo = 31%. The exercise condition was 45 minutes of walking on a treadmill at 70% to 85% maximum heart rate capacity, three times a week, for 16 weeks. The home-exercise group received the same instructions but was not supervised and had minimal contact with the research staff. The authors concluded that exercise's efficacy was comparable to that of medications. The supervised program was especially effective. The home program was slightly less effective but also comparable to medications. All treatments were more effective than the placebo.

A Cochrane review of 37 studies found that exercise was an effective treatment for depression (Cooney et al., 2013). It was as effective as psychotherapy in 7 trials, and as effective as medications in 4 trials. A systematic review of meta-analyses of experimental studies on exercise as a treatment for postpartum depression included 5 meta-analyses, with 2,419 participants (Marconcin et al., 2021). Exercise had a significant effect on postpartum depression, with a small effect size (SMD = –0.41; 95% CI: –0.50 to –0.32; p <0.001). When they eliminated overlapping cases, they found a moderate magnitude. They also found that exercise was more effective than psychosocial and psychological interventions, but also noted that exercise was used with other treatments in some of the studies, which they felt could account for the heterogeneity of findings.

Exercise for Pregnant and Postpartum Women

A meta-analysis of 12 studies examined the effects of exercise on mental health during pregnancy and postpartum (Poyatos-Leon et al., 2017). The combined sample was 932, with 471 in the intervention group and 461 in the control group. The exercises included walking, stretching and breathing, Pilates and yoga, and home programs. Frequency ranged from 1 to 5 days per week. They found an effect size of 0.41, which is small. However, in pooled analysis, the effect size was moderate (0.67) for mothers with postpartum depression at baseline and 0.29 for mothers who did not. They concluded that exercise during pregnancy and postpartum was a safe way to improve mental health and reduce postpartum depression. A narrative review of yoga and physical activity for pregnant and postpartum women found that it was an acceptable, feasible, and accessible alternative to standard mental healthcare (Eustis et al., 2019). They also noted that there were barriers to this type of treatment that need to be identified. Large-scale randomized trials were needed.

A study of 230 pregnant women examined the relationships between depressive symptoms, body image satisfaction, and exercise in the first, second, and third trimester of pregnancy, and at 6 weeks postpartum (Downs et al., 2008). If women had depressive symptoms and poor body image in early pregnancy, they were more likely to be depressed in late pregnancy. Exercise moderated these effects.

In a randomized trial, 62 mothers were enrolled in an 8-week program of exercise and parenting education, and 73 mothers were enrolled in education only (Norman et al., 2010). Mothers in the exercise/education group had significantly lower depression and higher well-being than the education-only group. Exercise reduced risk by 50%. In a sample of 80 women with postpartum depression at 6 weeks, women were assigned to exercise three times a week or receive standard care (Heh et al., 2008). Women who exercised were significantly less depressed at 5 months than the standard-care group.

A randomized trial of 38 women with postpartum depression found that exercise did not decrease depression, but it did increase self-efficacy (Daley et al., 2008).

Twelve hundred and twenty women from North Carolina were enrolled in a study in the third trimester of pregnancy (Demissie et al., 2011a). The researchers investigated the impact of moderate to vigorous activity on depressive symptoms. They assessed past-week physical activity at 17 to 22 weeks' gestation, and depressive symptoms at 24 to 29 weeks' gestation. Women who engaged in moderate to vigorous physical activity were half as likely to be depressed as women reporting lower levels of activity.

A meta-analysis of 6 trials with pregnant women found that exercise significantly reduced depression scores compared to women in the control conditions (Daley et al., 2015). The authors concluded that there was "some evidence" that exercise reduced depression in pregnancy, but the data were limited. Even with limited data, given exercise's other benefits, it seems a low-risk intervention to offer to pregnant women who are depressed or are at risk.

A review of 76 systematic reviews and meta-analyses found strong evidence that moderate-intensity exercise reduced gestational weight gain, gestational diabetes, and postpartum depression (Di Pietro et al., 2019). Exercise also reduced the risk for preeclampsia, gestational hypertension, and prenatal anxiety. The authors' primary focus was health conditions, such as hypertension and diabetes mellitus. However, they also assessed depression and anxiety and found that 30 minutes of moderate-intensity exercise, 3 to 5 times a week, for 4 weeks to 6 months, reduced depression.

Although the individual studies had positive results, a recent review noted that studies on exercise and depression in perinatal women have been limited by small samples, lack of comparison groups that control for time and other depression treatments (Reza et al., 2018). Similarly, a recent meta-analysis was also cautious (Carter et al., 2019). They examined 18 trials and found a moderate effect size of exercise in reducing depression in postpartum women up to 52 weeks. However, because of the heterogeneity of the studies, studies with high risk of bias were eliminated. When this was accounted for, the effect size was small. They found that exercise interventions were more effective for women with a history of depression or with depressive symptoms; targeted intervention or prevention was best. Most of the studies used aerobic exercise or coaching, but most were of poor quality. The authors were cautious about recommending exercise as an intervention until better studies existed. Nevertheless, they concluded that exercise as an intervention holds promise. Three of the studies reviewed earlier were included in this review.

Barriers to Exercise

Compliance can be an issue with exercise as an intervention. A small study randomized 24 inner-city women with postpartum depression to exercise vs. control groups (Forsyth et al., 2017). The women were living in Stoke-on-Trent in the UK, which was ranked in the bottom 5% nationally for poverty. They found no difference between the groups. Focus group data revealed that the women viewed exercise positively but had problems doing it. The exercises included pram (stroller) walking, exercising in a facility, or exercising at home. Barriers included lack of time or motivation, transportation, and adverse weather. None of the participants were exercisers before the study but were referred by a physician to be in the study.

A qualitative study included 21 structured interviews with British mothers who reported barriers to exercise as a treatment for depression that were physical, practical, and psychological (Pritchett et al., 2017). The 21 interviews were nested within a randomized trial. All the mothers had either depression or depression and anxiety. They also found ways to overcome barriers to exercise. Once they were able to exercise, mothers reported that it improved their sense of self, which had deteriorated while they were depressed.

The authors recommended that health professionals describe why exercise would help mothers who are reluctant and assist them in overcoming possible guilt because it benefits them and their infants (Pritchett et al., 2017). Walking was popular. Mothers identified fatigue, self-isolation, lack of motivation and inertia, worry about guilt if they failed, and guilt that they were taking time for themselves as barriers. Lack of childcare was another barrier. Self-criticism was common as they compared themselves to how they were pre-pregnancy. Eventually, mothers overcame barriers and incorporated exercise into their lives. They described gaining confidence and a sense of freedom from exercise. Mothers also liked using exercise to treat their depression since they did not need to tell others that they were depressed. In addition, they considered exercise a natural treatment.

Exercise Type

The early studies of exercise and depression all used aerobic exercise. More recent studies have incorporated other modalities. A review of 52 studies ($N = 131,406$) found that exercise only, and not exercise combined with another intervention, reduced prenatal depression. Supervised exercise had the greatest effect (Davenport et al., 2018). They suggested that women needed to exercise at least 150 minutes/week of moderate-intensity exercise, such as brisk walking, water aerobics, stationary cycling, and resistance training, to achieve a moderate effect size in reducing severity of prenatal depression. There was a dose-response effect for exercise: more exercise led to a greater reduction in symptoms. Exercise alone decreased prenatal depression by 67%. Prenatal exercise did not lower the risk for postpartum depression or anxiety, nor did it lessen severity. This suggests that exercise needs to continue into the postpartum period.

A study compared resistance training to flexibility training for a group of 60 postpartum women (LeCheminant et al., 2014). Resistance training twice a week significantly decreased depressive symptoms. There was no significant change for flexibility or waitlist conditions. Twenty-eight women from Taiwan participated in a yoga and Pilates program for 12 weeks at 2 to 6 months postpartum (Ko et al., 2013). Women with severe depression had a significant reduction in symptoms.

Other researchers examined yoga as a treatment for postpartum depression (Buttner et al., 2015). The researchers randomized 57 depressed women (Hamilton Depression Rating Scale >12) to either yoga or wait-list conditions. Women in the yoga group attended classes twice a week for 8 weeks. At the end of the trial, women in both groups had improved, but women in the yoga group had significantly improved depression, anxiety, and health-related quality of life than women in the wait-list condition, with large effect sizes. They noted that yoga is a promising integrative treatment for perinatal depression.

A review of 17 studies of postpartum depression and exercise found that leisure-time physical activity decreased postpartum depressive symptoms (Teychenne & York, 2013). The fact that exercise is defined as "leisure-time activity" might be key to understanding these findings. The study of 550 women in North Carolina found that if activity is fun, it lowers inflammation. If the activity is not fun (such as exercise that takes place as part of a job or caregiving), it increases inflammation (Demissie et al., 2011b).

Exercise and Breastfeeding

Although exercise offers many benefits, mothers may be concerned that it will negatively impact breastfeeding. Studies have generally found that exercise had no negative effects on breastfeeding (Amorin et al., 2007). An Australian study of 587 new mothers examined the relationship between mothers' exercise, initiation and duration of breastfeeding, and exercise's effect on infant growth (Su et al., 2007). At 6 to 12 months, exercise had not decreased breastfeeding duration. At 12 months, exercise had no significant impact on infants' growth. Researchers concluded exercise is safe for breastfeeding mothers and important for maintaining health.

A more specific question regarding exercise and breastfeeding is whether exercise causes lactic acid to build up in mothers' milk. In a study of 12 women, milk and blood samples were taken after a non-exercise session, after maximal exercise, and after a session that was 20% below the maximal range (Quinn & Carey, 1999). They found that in women with an adequate caloric intake, moderate exercise neither increased lactic acid in breastmilk nor caused babies to reject it. When women exercised in the "hard" range (using the perceived-exertion scale), lactic acid increased. The authors recommended exercise in a moderate range.

A narrative review found that lactic acid can build in milk after extreme exercise but that mild to moderate exercise does not cause lactic acid to accumulate (Mortensen & Kam, 2012). More sensitive measures found increased lactic acid after moderate exercise, but it did not influence infants' acceptance of the milk. Further, moderate exercise did not alter immune qualities in the milk, such as sIgA, lactoferrin, and lysozyme. Nor did it influence the long-chain polyunsaturated fatty acids in breastmilk.

Exercise Is Anti-Inflammatory

Exercise lowers inflammation, which is why it helps with depression. People who exercise have lower inflammatory biomarkers than people who are sedentary (Kiecolt-Glaser et al., 2015). Chronic inflammation affects the body's composition and metabolism in several ways, including the loss of body protein and the accretion of fat (Roubenoff, 2003). For example, cachexia, or loss of lean muscle mass, is at least partially mediated by the proinflammatory cytokines IL-1β, IL-6, and TNF-α. Exercise can reverse these inflammatory-mediated changes.

Initially, exercise acts as an acute physical stressor and raises IL-6 and TNF-α. Over a longer period, however, as exercise becomes a regular habit, it lowers inflammation. Older adults, for example, are one group with higher levels of proinflammatory cytokines, since levels naturally increase as we age. Indeed, researchers hypothesize that this age-related rise in inflammation creates vulnerability to diseases, such as heart disease, cancer, and Alzheimer's (Kiecolt-Glaser et al., 2007). Because of this increased vulnerability of older adults, they are frequently the population of choice for studies on exercise, depression, and inflammation. The results of these studies are helpful for understanding the mechanism underlying exercise's impact on depression.

A study of adults, ages 60 to 90, tested the effects of physical activity on perceived stress, mood, and quality of life (Starkweather, 2007). The researchers also assessed serum

IL-6 and cortisol. The patients ($N = 10$) assigned to the exercise group were instructed to walk for 30 minutes, 5 times a week, for the 10-week study. The control group were 10 older adults who were not engaging in physical activity. After the 10-week exercise intervention, the subjects had significantly lower stress on the Perceived Stress Scale, improved mood and quality of life, and a significant decrease in serum IL-6. They reported better physical functioning, more vitality, better mental health, and less bodily pain than the non-exercising group.

Exercise also had a positive effect on wound healing, and this is an indirect measure of systemic inflammation (Emery et al., 2005). In this study, participants were randomized into exercise and control conditions and were given a punch biopsy to monitor rate of wound healing. Exercise 1 hour a day, 3 days a week, lowered perceived stress and improved wound healing. For the exercise group, wounds healed in 29 days. In the control group, it took 38 days. This study is of interest because high stress or hostility impairs wound healing and increases systemic inflammation (Kiecolt-Glaser et al., 2005). High inflammation impairs wound healing because proinflammatory cytokines are systemic in the plasma and not at the wound site, where they belong. The Emery et al. (2005) study indicates that exercise improves wound healing by diverting circulating cytokines to the wound site.

General fitness also lowers inflammation (Hamer & Steptoe, 2007). The sample were 207 men and women from London. Participants whose systolic blood pressure increased when stressed in the lab also had an increase in inflammation. The TNF-α response to stress was 5 times greater in the low-fitness vs. the high-fitness group. Participants who were physically fit had a lower inflammation response when under stress, which likely protected them from both depression and chronic disease.

Clinical Takeaways

- Exercise effectively treats depression—alone or in combination with other treatments—and has no negative effect on breastfeeding.
- The major challenge with exercise is getting depressed mothers to do it, because it is often the last thing they feel like doing. However, mothers may be motivated to try when they realize that it's an effective alternative to medications.
- Blumenthal et al.'s (2007) study found a slightly higher remission in the supervised vs. at-home exercise. Compliance rates were likely higher because participants knew people expected them to show up to exercise. The supervised program also provided social support. Getting a group of mothers together to exercise can help with their depression and break their sense of isolation.
- Mothers should aim for 150 minutes of exercise per week.

11 Bright Light Therapy

Some people dread the change of seasons. Shorter, darker days mean fatigue, oversleeping, overeating, and having a general sense of malaise: a pattern known as seasonal affective disorder (SAD) (Sullivan & Payne, 2007). Symptoms include depression, lethargy, difficulty waking, impaired concentration, lack of interest in social activities, and craving carbohydrates, which can lead to winter weight gain (National Alliance on Mental Illness (NAMI), 2007). In industrialized countries, most people are exposed to bright light (>1,000 lux) only about an hour a day. If a person is not susceptible to seasonal depression, this is not a problem. If, however, someone is susceptible, it can be (Crowley & Youngstedt, 2012). Patients with SAD were the first to use light as a treatment for depression. Researchers have demonstrated that it is very effective.

KEY FINDINGS

- Bright light therapy has a long track record of effectively treating depression. It can be added to other modalities.
- Morning light exposure appears to be most effective. Dawn simulation can be a viable alternative for a new mother who does not have time to sit in front of a light box every day.
- Ten thousand lux is the intensity most often used in studies, but some dimmer lights have been effective.

Bright light therapy effectively treats seasonal affective disorder in non-postpartum samples, and the response is often within days (National Alliance on Mental Illness (NAMI), 2007). An expert panel for the American Psychiatric Association concluded that bright light therapy effectively treats both seasonal and non-seasonal depression, with results comparable to antidepressants (Golden et al., 2005). Light therapy can also treat perinatal depression (Oren et al., 2002; Terman & Terman, 2005).

Light Therapy in Pregnant and Postpartum Women

To date, only a few studies of bright light therapy have specifically included pregnant and postpartum women. Bright light alleviated depression in two case studies of new mothers who became depressed after the birth of their babies (Corral et al., 2000). These mothers refused antidepressants but agreed to a trial of bright light therapy. Both responded to bright light therapy and had significantly lower rates of depressive symptoms after treatment.

DOI: 10.4324/9781003405092-13

A study included 27 German pregnant women with non-seasonal major depression who were randomized into bright light (7,000 lux) or 70 lux dim red light for 1 hour per day in the morning for 5 weeks (Wirz-Justice et al., 2017). At 5 weeks, women in the bright light group had a 4-point drop on the Hamilton Depression Rating Scale, which impressed the authors, who noted that a 2-point drop is typical in antidepressant studies.

Another randomized trial included 22 women with EPDS scores >12. Eleven were assigned to bright light (10,000 lux), and 11 to dim light (19 lux) (Garbazza et al., 2022). They used light in the morning for 30 minutes a day. Women in the bright light group achieved 73% remission (improvement of 50% or greater) compared to 27% in the dim light group. In addition, the women in the bright light group had a greater reduction in symptoms across the follow-up period. There were no side effects in either group.

Thirty pregnant or postpartum women with major depression were assigned to bright light (10,000 lux) or placebo light (<500 lux) (Donmez et al., 2022). The light was used for 45 minutes every morning for 3 weeks. At 3 weeks, there was a 75% response rate with bright light compared to 18% for the placebo. The remission rates were 42% vs. 0%. There was no difference between the groups in adverse effects.

Bright light therapy was also used in a study of mothers with babies in the NICU (Ball et al., 2012). In addition to the normal stresses associated with having a baby in the NICU, NICUs had low light levels, which desynchronizes circadian rhythms. The authors conducted a pilot study with 30 mothers, randomizing 15 mothers to receive 3 weeks of bright light therapy. Seventy-three percent of the mothers were African American, with a mean age of 26. The light in the NICU was <10 lux bedside, and 100 lux in the lobby. The design called for mothers using a light visor, and the adherence rate was approximately 88%. Mothers in the experimental group had lower levels of depression, less fatigue, and improved health-related quality of life. Their sleep quality was also better. None of the between-group differences were statistically significant due to the small sample size, but they were clinically significant. Further, the effect sizes ranged from small to large.

According to Crowley and Youngstedt (2012), perinatal women may be particularly vulnerable to the lack of light exposure. At the end of pregnancy, they may be restricted in their mobility and therefore not spend as much time outside. After the baby is born, they may also spend more time indoors, and sleep during the day. Both can desynchronize circadian rhythms, increasing the risk for depression.

Light Intensity, Duration, and Timing of Light Exposure

There are several characteristics of light related to its effectiveness as a treatment. These characteristics include light intensity, duration, and timing of light exposure.

Intensity

Researchers have investigated a wide range of light intensities, and several appear effective. Light intensity is measured in lux, which is brightness by proximity. Lights at closer distances have a higher lux than the same light that is further away.

Ten thousand lux was traditionally considered most effective. At this level of intensity, 30 to 40 minutes of exposure is sufficient. Two studies with light exposures of 30 to 40 minutes at 10,000 lux achieved a 75% remission rate in depression. It took 2 hours to achieve similar remission rates at 2,500 lux, and in some cases, even with longer exposure, lower-intensity lights were not effective (Terman & Terman, 2005). Longer exposure times mean that patients are less likely to comply. This may particularly be true for mothers of young children, who probably won't find it practical to sit in front of a light box for 2 or 3 hours.

However, a study used a Litebook LED (1,350 lux) for 30 minutes and found that that amount of light significantly lowered depression scores compared to a placebo light (Desan et al., 2007). This was a small trial (*N* = 23), and patients were assessed after 1, 2, 3, and 4 weeks of treatment. By 4 weeks, 57% of patients in the LED condition were in remission compared to 11% of patients in the control group. The authors speculated that this lower-intensity light worked because it was in the 450 to 480 nanometer range, and that melatonin rhythms were best shifted by those wavelengths. Because of this concentration in short wavelengths, even lower-intensity light might prove as effective as brighter light boxes while using smaller, more convenient devices.

A more recent study randomized 67 depressed pregnant women to either 9,000 lux or dim red light therapy (100 lux) (Bais et al., 2020). Participants used the lights for 6 weeks for 30 minutes upon awakening. Depression in the bright light group dropped by 41% to 53%. For women in the dim light group, depression dropped by 51% to 67%. Both treatments appeared effective at impressive rates. The authors suggest further investigation to find out why.

Timing

Morning bright light is generally more successful than light exposure later in the day. In their review of 25 studies, Terman and Terman (2005) found significantly higher remission rates with morning exposure (53%) compared with mid-day (32%) and evening (38%). One exception to the use of morning light is in patients with bipolar disorder. Morning light exposure increases risk for a manic episode. For these patients, timing light exposure to later in the day and having them continue on their medications during light treatment addresses these concerns (National Alliance on Mental Illness (NAMI), 2007; Terman & Terman, 2005).

Dawn Simulation

Because of the effectiveness of morning light exposure, a variant to standard light therapy has been added to the repertoire of possible treatments: dawn simulation. As the name implies, *dawn simulation* refers to a light that comes on before a patient is awake and gradually increases in intensity over a period of 15 to 90 minutes (the length can be tailored to individual preference). The advantage to this treatment is that it does not require sitting in front of a light box for an extended time, making it more practical for new mothers or mothers of young children. Some devices are both light boxes and dawn simulators.

Terman and Terman (2006) randomly assigned 99 adults with seasonal major depression to one of five treatment conditions. These included dawn simulation, dawn light pulse, post-awakening bright light therapy (30 minutes at 10,000 lux), negative air ionization at high flow rate, and ionization at low flow rate. After three weeks of treatment, patients who received bright light therapy (57%) and dawn simulation (50%) had the greatest improvement in symptoms. They concluded that bright light therapy was the most effective. However, if there are problems with non-compliance or non-response, dawn simulation or dawn pulse are viable alternatives.

Why Light Is Effective

Researchers have proposed several possible mechanisms for why bright light alleviates depression. Most have to do with modifying the internal circadian clock. Our circadian rhythms, or daily patterns of sleep and arousal, are regulated by the pineal gland, which secretes melatonin. The suprachiasmatic nucleus of the hypothalamus regulates synthesis of melatonin (Erman, 2007). The pineal gland responds to light via light receptors in the retina. The superiority of morning light exposure is likely due to the diurnal variations in retinal photoreceptor sensitivity, with greater sensitivity to morning light. Indeed, exposure to evening light can lead to insomnia and hyperactivation in some people (National Alliance on Mental Illness (NAMI), 2007; Terman & Terman, 2005).

A theory about why dawn simulation works is because of its impact on the early dawn interval, when melatonin levels wane and core body temperature rises (Terman, 2006). The early dawn interval is when circadian rhythms are most susceptible to light-elicited phase advances. According to this theory, depression is more likely to be triggered when it is still dark outdoors in the early dawn interval.

Inflammation may be involved as well. Lam and colleagues (2004) hypothesized that during winter, proinflammatory cytokines increase in patients with seasonal depression. In a study of 15 patients and a matched group of normal controls, those with seasonal affective disorder had significantly higher levels of IL-6. After 2 weeks of bright light therapy, symptoms improved, and 64% of patients had at least a 50% reduction in depressive symptoms. However, light therapy did not lower inflammation after 2 weeks. The authors concluded that seasonal depression involves activation of the immune-inflammatory system, which is not immediately altered by light therapy (Leu et al., 2001).

Safety Issues

Because light boxes appear to be simple, patients often consider assembling a unit themselves. Clinicians generally recommend that patients not use homemade devices, for several reasons. First, it is difficult for consumers to find lights that are sufficiently bright enough to generate a therapeutic effect. Second, some patients have experienced excessive irradiation and corneal or eyelid burns with homemade devices. Finally, homemade devices often use incandescent lights, which are not recommended because 90% of light output from incandescent bulbs is on the infrared end of the spectrum. Not only can infrared exposure at high intensity burn the lens, cornea, and retina, but it is also on the wrong end of the color spectrum for a therapeutic effect (Terman & Terman, 2005). The National Alliance on Mental Illness (2007) recommends bulbs with a color temperature between 3,000 and 6,500 degrees Kelvin and are in the white-to-blue range of the color spectrum. These do not harm patients' eyes.

Ultraviolet (UV) can also damage eyes. The National Alliance on Mental Illness (2007) recommends light boxes with a UV filter. Patients wanting to try light therapy should use a lighting apparatus from a reputable dealer. Many are available for a reasonable price on Amazon.

Clinical Takeaways

- Bright light therapy is a generally safe, well-tolerated treatment option for perinatal depression. It is also breastfeeding-friendly and can be safely used during pregnancy.
- Mothers often feel better quickly. If mothers are on antidepressants, bright light and exercise can help mothers improve in the 4 to 6 weeks it takes for antidepressants to be effective.
- Quality lightboxes are available online and are more affordable than ever (ranging from $19 to $50 USD).

12 Emerging CAM Treatments

Other CAM treatments that have been effective in the general population are now being used in perinatal women. These approaches are promising and appear effective for treating even severe depression. These modalities include acupuncture, transcranial direct current stimulation (tDCS), and repetitive transcranial magnetic stimulation (rTMS).

KEY FINDINGS

- Acupuncture is more effective in treating perinatal depression than sham acupuncture or massage. Acupuncture also produces changes in the brain, which may affect symptoms.
- tDCS and rTMS both use mild electrical stimulation, repeated over several sessions, to treat depression and PTSD. Both are non-invasive and do not require anesthesia. Both have Level A (definite efficacy) ratings from health organizations in Europe and the US.

Acupuncture

Acupuncture has been used to treat major depression and PTSD in a number of studies (Bai et al., 2013; Kim, Heo, et al., 2013). A review of 52 systematic reviews or meta-analyses found that acupuncture was effective for treating headaches and appears promising for anxiety, sleep disturbances, depression, and chronic pain (Lee et al., 2012). Acupuncture helped alleviate symptoms in two studies of major depression in pregnant women (Manber et al., 2004; Manber et al., 2010). The response rate was 69% in the first study for acupuncture, 47% for sham acupuncture, and 32% for massage, with 20 pregnant women in each group. Sham acupuncture involves using small metal "needles" that look like acupuncture needles and appear to puncture the skin but do not.

In the second study, 150 pregnant women with major depression were also randomized to treatment to acupuncture specific for depression, acupuncture not specific for depression, and massage groups (Manber et al., 2010). In both acupuncture groups, practitioners avoided points that should not be used with pregnant women because they could start labor contractions. The remission rates were 63% for acupuncture specific for depression, 44% for acupuncture not specific for depression, and 38% for massage.

A recent review included 887 patients with postpartum depression from 12 randomized trials (Tong et al., 2019). Of these, 443 were treated with acupuncture and 444 were in control groups. Patients in the treatment group had significantly better scores on the Hamilton Depression Rating Scale and Edinburgh Postnatal Depression Scale than

DOI: 10.4324/9781003405092-14

those in control groups. However, the authors were circumspect regarding their findings. The control groups in the 12 studies all had active treatments: 9 to 12 used medications, 1 had therapy, 2 used Traditional Chinese Medicine, and 1 used massage. In addition, the acupuncture studies did not include acupuncture alone: 3 also included psychological interventions, and 3 included Traditional Chinese Medicine. When acupuncture alone was used, it made no significant difference in depression scores.

In a meta-analysis of 8 studies on acupuncture and postpartum depression, the authors found that acupuncture lowered scores on the Hamilton Depression Rating Scale (HAM-D) but did not lower scores on the EPDS or change clinical responses (Li et al., 2019). The finding on the HAM-D vs. EPDS is surprising in that the HAM-D is a more stringent scale. They noted that the sample sizes were small in the studies, and there was heterogeneity in findings.

Another review included 15 studies of acupuncture and Chinese herbal medicine to treat postpartum depression that were included in English and Chinese databases (Yang et al., 2018). They found that the evidence was low-quality (per the Cochrane risk-of-bias tool). But when acupuncture and Chinese herbal medicine were used alone or combined with antidepressants, they reduced depression symptoms on the EPDS compared to a placebo or antidepressants. There was no significant difference between acupuncture and antidepressants, and adverse effects were rare.

The mechanism by which acupuncture influences mental health is unclear. It may be anti-inflammatory (Tong et al., 2019). It may also influence the function of specific brain regions, such as the amygdala. A recent study of 52 women with postpartum depression (22 of whom had acupuncture) and 24 non-depressed controls found that women with postpartum depression had decreased gray matter volume in sub-regions of the amygdala (left and right lateral) compared to the healthy postpartum women (Huang et al., 2023). The HAM-D scores improved for the depressed women after being treated with acupuncture, and the gray matter volume marginally improved. The treated women also showed a significantly enhanced resting-state functional magnetic resonance imaging (fMRI). The authors concluded that acupuncture may improve symptoms because it changes the amygdala sub-region structure and the functional connections of brain areas that process negative emotions. fMRI can help researchers examine these changes, which may be the central mechanism by which acupuncture improves mental health.

Transcranial Direct Current Stimulation (tDCS) and Repetitive Transcranial Magnetic Stimulation (rTMS)

Two gentle brain-stimulation techniques are also showing promising results. Both techniques, tDCS and rTMS, are non-invasive, do not require anesthesia, and have few side effects. When there are side effects, they are mild and temporary. Both techniques work by affecting brain function and activity. rTMS is a neuro*modulator*, which stimulates nerves to provide a natural biological response. tDCS is a neuro*stimulator*, which involves direct application of electrodes to the brain, spinal cord, or peripheral nerves. A TENS unit (transcutaneous electrical nerve stimulator), a device to help with chronic pain, is an example of a neurostimulator.

These treatments should not be confused with electroconvulsive therapy (ECT), which requires anesthesia and uses sufficient current to provoke a seizure. ECT is not a gentle technique and can lead to memory loss and confusion.

Repetitive Transcranial Magnetic Stimulation

Repetitive transcranial magnetic stimulation (rTMS) uses gentle magnetic pulse. It stimulates the brain by passing electrical current through a magnetic coil, which creates a magnetic field over the scalp. The tiny currents stimulate neuronal activity, and it stimulates the right and left dorsolateral prefrontal cortex. Repetitive transcranial magnetic stimulation has effectively treated depression, OCD, and PTSD, as well as pain, stroke, and several diseases. There is much research to support this modality, and it has been FDA-cleared for treating depression. Recent European evidence-based guidelines found rTMS effective at Level A (definite efficacy) or Level B (probable efficacy) for these conditions (Lefaucheur et al., 2020).

A consensus statement included 118 articles plus expert opinion on rTMS for treating major depression (McClintock et al., 2018). Multiple randomized controlled trials supported the safety and efficacy of rTMS as an antidepressant therapy. The authors wrote this statement on behalf of the National Network of Depression Centers rTMS Task Force and the American Psychiatric Association's Council on Research Task Force on Novel Biomarkers and Treatments.

A small study used repetitive transcranial magnetic stimulation to treat 6 postpartum women with depression (Cox et al., 2020). The women received 20 sessions of 10 Hertz rTMS over the left dorsolateral prefrontal cortex over 4 weeks. Researchers measured depression, anxiety, and breastfeeding practices at baseline, and at 3 and 6 months postpartum. There was no control group, which does not account for the placebo effect. Depression and anxiety scores declined over the 4-week treatment period. Depression was lower at 3 and 6 months. Of the six patients, 4 achieved remission.

A review of 14 studies ($N = 884$ participants) found that rTMS reduced scores on the HAM-D and EPDS and improved cognitive function in patients with postpartum depression (Peng et al., 2020). They included studies from both English and Chinese databases. The studies were all randomized trials and were excluded if they did not have either a control group or a group who received sham treatment.

In a functional imaging study, 32 women with postpartum depression were compared with 32 age-matched healthy controls (Zhang, Mu, et al., 2022). They found that women with postpartum depression had reduced voxel-mirrored homotopic connectivity in the amygdala, insula, and medial frontal gyrus of the brain compared to healthy volunteers. These regions renormalized after rTMS. In addition, increased connectivity between the right and left insula was correlated with improved EPDS scores. They concluded that intrinsic functional architecture of the interhemispheric communication was disrupted in postpartum depression, which they believed provided evidence for the pathophysiological mechanisms and effects of rTMS.

Transcranial Direct Current Stimulation

Transcranial direct current stimulation (tDCS) involves sending a weak electrical current across the brain via electrodes on either side of the head, which modulates brain activity in cognitive and motor domains. tDCS has been used to effectively treat depression, and recent evidence-based guidelines rate the evidence as Level A: definitely effective for depression (Fregni et al., 2021). A review of 12 randomized, sham-controlled trials ($N = 251$ sham group; 204 treatment) found that combining tDCS with medication significantly lowered depression scores in depressed adults (Wang et al., 2021). tDCS and medication were more effective than sham treatments. As a monotreatment, or combined with psychotherapy, tDCS was effective.

A pilot randomized trial included 16 depressed pregnant women who had refused antidepressants. Treatment involved 2 mAmp direct current to the dorsolateral prefrontal cortex over 30 minutes. The treatment took place 5 times a week for 3 weeks. The sham treatment turned off the current after 30 seconds. At 4 weeks postpartum, 75% of the treatment group was in remission vs. 13% of the sham treatment group.

A review of 7 studies, with 33 perinatal women, found that there were no adverse effects for either mother or child with tDCS (Laurin et al., 2022). They noted that the results are encouraging, but that larger studies need to be conducted. They also presented three case studies: a pregnant woman with type-2 bipolar depression, a pregnant woman with PTSD, and a breastfeeding woman with postpartum depression. All improved with treatment and reported only minor side effects. There were no adverse effects on the infant.

Clinical Takeaways

- Acupuncture has effectively treated major depression in pregnant and postpartum women. However, it is often combined with Traditional Chinese Medicine or antidepressants. It may work as a monotherapy, but that has not been well-established.
- Repetitive transcranial stimulation (rTMS) has an evidence base supporting its use in the general population. Perinatal studies have been promising.
- Transcranial direct current stimulation (tDCS) also effectively treats depression and involves weak current across the brain.
- Both treatments are gentle and should not be confused with electroconvulsive therapy (ECT). ECT requires anesthesia and can cause memory loss and confusion. The weaker current in rTMS and tDCS treats depression without those negative side effects.
- It may be challenging to find a provider in your community, but all these treatments are becoming more widely available.

Section III

Community Interventions

13 Social Support
The Foundation to Community Support

Many practitioners underestimate the important of social support, thinking it is nice but not critical. We now know that that is simply not true; human beings need relationships with others. Social support alters our physiology and changes brain activity. Because of its powerful physiological effects, social support can prevent and even treat depression. Social support is also anti-inflammatory, which explains why it prevents so many diseases. A meta-analysis of 41 studies ($N = 73,037$) found that social support and social integration significantly lowered levels of inflammation (Uchino et al., 2018). In short, people with social support live longer and happier lives.

KEY FINDINGS

- Social support is important during all stages of life. People with social support lead happier, healthier lives. Social support also helps new mothers navigate the perinatal period.
- The most important type of support is responsive. When the mothers' thoughts, feelings, and needs are considered, other types of support become more effective. Without responsive support, "supportive actions" have a negative effect and feel like judgment, coercion, or control.
- It is more accurate to measure mothers' perceived support than task-based support in relation to depression.

As an intervention, social support is amenable to mothers. In a wide variety of cultures, depressed mothers prefer talking with someone rather than taking medications (Dennis & Chung-Lee, 2006). Support can happen in families, in informal community settings interventions, or as part of psychotherapy. In a qualitative study of 41 Canadian new mothers, partners, friends, family, other mothers, and healthcare providers were important sources of support that helped women recover from postpartum depression (Letourneau et al., 2007). In this study, practical and informational support were the most helpful types. Affirmation worked best when it came from other mothers who had been depressed. In the beginning, mothers preferred one-on-one to group or telephone support. However, as they recovered, group support helped.

Social support also has a powerful effect on the brain. A recent Chinese study examined functional connectivity strength between brain regions. When functional connectivity strength is high, depression risk increases. Social support lowers risk of depression and anxiety by mediating cerebellum functional connectivity strength (Cheng et al., 2022). This study examined women using resting-state functional magnetic imaging resonance

DOI: 10.4324/9781003405092-16

(fMRI): 45 women with postpartum depression, 31 women with depression and anxiety, 62 control volunteers. Perceived social support was related to lower scores on the EPDS and the Beck Anxiety Inventory (BAI), which corresponded to lower functional connectivity strength. Depressed women had higher functional connectivity strength in the right parahippocampus and the left paracentral lobule. Women with anxiety had higher functional connectivity in the left ventrolateral prefrontal cortex. Perceived social support mediated the influence of the functional connectivity strength in the right cerebellum posterior lobe on depression and anxiety symptoms. The authors noted that social support is important for maintaining mental health in postpartum women.

Support Lowers the Risk for Depression

The Fragile Families and Child Well-Being Study, a study of 4,900 births from 75 US hospitals, found that life stress increased risk for postpartum depression (Reid & Taylor, 2015). Partner, friend, and family support lowered risk for all women regardless of family type. For disadvantaged mothers, support is even more important, as most face significant life stress. A Canadian study of refugees and asylum seekers found that social support from family, friends, church, work, or school increased resilience and lowered depression risk in women who had experienced many lifetime adversities (Gagnon & Stewart, 2014).

Social support helps even under extreme circumstances. A study from Thailand compared 233 migrants and 218 refugees on the Thai/Myanmar border (Fellmeth et al., 2021). The migrants were those who crossed the Thai border seeking work. They supported themselves (albeit at a low level) and had freedom of movement. The refugees were in camps in Thailand. They had food and shelter but had very limited freedom of movement and were not allowed to seek employment. Fellmeth et al. (2021) found that 39% of migrants and 47% of refugees had perinatal depression diagnosed via structured clinical interview. These numbers included women with mild depression. Interestingly, 89% of migrants reported sufficient support, and 86% had supportive partners. In contrast, 49% of refugees reported sufficient support, and 53% had supportive partners. Received support significantly lowered depression in migrant women. If refugee women believed their support was insufficient, their risk for depression increased by 90%. Each increase in received support reduced their risk for depression by 20%. For both groups, history of depression and trauma increased the risk for depression.

COVID-19 gave researchers another opportunity to study the effect of support under extreme circumstances (Gildner et al., 2021). This study included 971 pregnant American women. If they gave birth later in the pandemic, they had instrumental support with housework and childcare, which lowered their risk for depression. The sample was educated and affluent: 85% had a bachelor's degree or higher, and 61% made over $100,000 per year. The overall depression rates were 11% (>13 on the EPDS). The hypothesis was that early in the pandemic, there was less social support because of stay-at-home orders. When those requirements were loosened, social support was more available.

A review from Thailand examined 13 studies of programs designed to prevent postpartum depression in adolescents (Sangsawang et al., 2019). Six of 13 studies reported positive results from their interventions. Most studies included American ethnic minorities, such as American Indians, Blacks, or Hispanics. These studies included two types of psychotherapy (cognitive-behavioral therapy and interpersonal psychotherapy), three community interventions (home visiting, prenatal and postpartum education), and infant massage. They could not identify which type was most effective but recommended them all as possible methods to prevent postpartum depression in teens.

Conversely, lack of support increased the risk of depression by 4.6 times in an Australian study of 1,070 women (Ramakrishna et al., 2019). Low support tripled depression risk in 596 mothers from Northern Ethiopia, as did lack of a partner due to death, divorce, or never marrying (Shitu et al., 2019).

What Is Effective Support?

Social support is obviously important. The next issue is defining what it is. Support can take many forms. Information at just the right time. Reassurance that things are going well or empathy when they are not. Practical help such as picking up groceries, doing the dishes, or watching the baby so the mother can take a shower. All these are important, but something that looks like support to observers may not be experienced as support by mothers—and that's what counts. Support is more than just having people around, or even people doing things for mothers. It needs to provide help *for that mother*.

To reiterate, within the construct of social support, there are two main components: the supportive action and mothers' *perception* of the action. In other words, did it feel like support to her? Take for example cleaning someone's home. Generally speaking, that is a kind act. Doing it for a new mother allows her to rest and focus on her baby. However, what if the mother feels judged, where there is a silent, or even spoken, question of, "Why aren't you doing this yourself?" or "I didn't have help after I had a baby. You're lucky." In this context, "help" does not feel good and can even make mothers feel judged and "lazy."

A recent study on breastfeeding support gives insight into these nuances. Davidson and Ollerton (2020) reviewed 8 articles on fathers' support for breastfeeding. Their findings get at the fundamental structure of support: action and perception of the action. When fathers offered help and encouragement, breastfeeding initiation increased, but women sometimes had negative views of "help and encouragement."

Responsiveness was the most effective kind of support and included being sensitive to women's needs, respecting their decisions, and promoting self-efficacy. If fathers took mothers' needs seriously and mothers and fathers acted together as a team, breastfeeding initiation, exclusivity, and duration increased. When fathers offered knowledge, help, and encouragement without responsiveness, breastfeeding duration decreased. With responsiveness, women felt understood, validated, and cared for. Without responsiveness, practical support meant that they are not self-sufficient, and encouragement felt like coercion to breastfeed or meet impossible breastfeeding goals. This study was specific to fathers' support for breastfeeding, but the principles it revealed are relevant to anyone providing support to new mothers. *Responsiveness to the mothers' needs is the most important thing. Without it, any other types of "support" may do more harm than good.* This mother described how many people wanted to help her but inadvertently undermined her.

> Everyone was really helping with the baby but me. They were too "supportive." I know my husband wouldn't want to think that. I felt like they were taking over everything. . . . I'm a very private person. I felt like everything was exposed.

Friends and family did not know how to help another depressed new mother. However, one friend provided effective support even though she did not fully understand.

> My friends didn't know what to do. They thought I had had a nervous breakdown. Many stayed away. Even now, many are surprised that I can still function. I had one friend who was very supportive and loving continually, even though she didn't understand. She brought meals, wrote little notes. She made no demands on my recovery. My mother-in-law and husband were helpful during that time too.

A study from rural Pakistan also contrasted mothers' perceived support with functional support over the first year postpartum (Hagaman et al., 2021). The sample included 780 women who were recruited over the last trimester of pregnancy and were assessed at 6 and 12 months postpartum. High and sustained social support, based on scores from the Multidimensional Scale of Perceived Social Support (MSPSS), decreased the risk of depression at 12 months. This was not true for scores on the Maternal Social Support Index (MSSI). The MSPSS measures *perceived support* from family and friends across multiple domains. The MSSI measures *task-based support* with 8 tasks (such as meal preparation). Perceived support was negatively correlated with depression, but task-based support (per the MSSI) was not. About 30% of the women in the sample had less than a primary education, and 45% experienced partner violence in the past year. High perceived support reduced the risk for depression at 12 months compared to low perceived support.

Clinical Takeaways

- Mothers' perception of support is the most important determinant of whether support will reduce their risk of depression. If they do not think the action supports them, it will not lower their risk of depression.
- Social support is not simply "nice." It causes dramatic physiological changes and lowers inflammation. Recent studies indicate that it may also change the brain.

14 Peer and Healthcare Provider Support

Community-based support is an important way for mothers to interpret, negotiate, and experience social norms of motherhood (Dennis & Chung-Lee, 2006). While social support can come from many informal sources, such as family members, friends, and community groups, the focus of this chapter is on formal community support programs. These can be delivered by peers or healthcare providers. The goal of these interventions is to lower rates of postpartum depression and ensure that mothers have access to services that they need.

KEY FINDINGS

- Peers and healthcare providers both provide postpartum support. However, reimbursement for services is important. Volunteer peers can provide excellent services, but paying them becomes an equity issue. Without pay, you limit the number of true peers in your program.
- Telephone support can be comparable to in-person and is a more cost-effective option. Digital self-help was also effective. Apps, so far, have not been effective.

Identity of the Supporter: Peer or Professional?

Providers of community support are either peers or professionals. Peer support can be more cost-effective but are often more time-intensive to train and support: there must be sufficient resources to train and supervise peers so they provide effective care and do not burn out. Peers can also have a high turnover rate, which increases costs for recruitment and training of new volunteers. Payment for peer supporters is also an equity issue (see next section). In contrast, healthcare provider support can be more "professional," can identify medical issues more quickly, and may have more authority with parents so that they listen to their recommendations. However, without personal experience, they may be less empathic (although this is not always true).

We struggle with the peer vs. professional balance in the lactation field. Some of the best lactation consultants I know started as peer supporters, and some of the worst are professionals. But there are excellent people in both groups. This section reviews studies on both peer and professional support as it relates to postpartum depression.

Peer Support

Leger and Letourneau (2015) noted that studies typically include four types of social support: informational, emotional, affirmational, and instrumental. Peer support provides a

DOI: 10.4324/9781003405092-17

fifth type: empathetic. They contrast this to emotional support, where there are expressions of concern and compassion, and affirmational support, which supports mothers' choices and behaviors. Empathetic support overlaps with these, but the main distinction is based on lived experience of postpartum depression.

O'Hara (2022) grappled with the issue of using peers to provide support. He asked how someone would go about identifying peers. Is someone a peer because they have also experienced postpartum depression? Or are they peers because of similar age, socioeconomic status, relationship status, cultural identity, and race/ethnicity? Does the nature of "peerness" matter in terms of an effective intervention (O'Hara, 2022)?

In their review, Leger and Letourneau (2015) found that the most effective programs were those where the volunteers matched the families in terms of demographics and experiences. Training is essential, and many good training manuals already exist. These manuals teach how volunteers can normalize an experience without minimizing it. Without training, volunteers may be unintentionally unsupportive.

The next important question is, How much training should they receive (Leger & Letourneau, 2015)? What are the essential qualities of peer support, and are they diminished when delivered in a structured intervention? Peers share their own experiences, model and offer hope for recovery. Peers can share their own experiences, but professionals are not supposed to. Interestingly, O'Hara (2022) is not in favor of peer support. Rather, he supports "lay interventionists," such as midwives and nurses, as they are already in the health system and can bill for their services. This raises a final question: How can peers be compensated for the work that they do? Is it fair to rely solely on volunteers? Volunteer vs. paid labor also becomes an equity issue, as many low-income women cannot dedicate the time necessary to provide good support without being paid for it. As we have found in the lactation field, it is often only the White middle-class women who can afford to work for free or with low pay. To ensure that lower-income women have access to peer support, supporters need to be paid. These are all important considerations when deciding whether to implement a peer-support program.

In a narrative review of 6 studies on peer support for postpartum depression, more than 80% of mothers were satisfied with the support they received (Leger & Letourneau, 2015). The volunteers enjoyed it too. Mothers cited "She listens" as a main point. They also appreciated practical support with childcare and household chores. However, in one study, about 10% of mothers reported that their peer minimized their problems, and 12% said their peer "talked too much." The volunteers sometimes felt overwhelmed with the needs of these mothers and families. They also found it difficult to provide support when they were unable to establish friendship bonds with mothers. Peers felt that there were many other areas where mothers needed help but they were not qualified to provide it. However, peers received satisfaction when they saw positive change, especially when these mothers had little support; peers knew they made a difference.

Leger and Letourneau (2015) recommended that volunteers receive training before they provide support and that they be asked about their ability to commit to the time required. Other recommendations included interventions targeted toward mothers' culture and circumstances. They noted that although the findings were mixed, peers can be an important part of the treatment team.

A recent review applied a realist methodology, which was tested against empirical data from 29 studies (22 interventions) on peer support for prenatal and postpartum mental health (McLeish et al., 2023). Three programs offered one-on-one support from a trained volunteer, one had a paid peer supporter, 11 offered in-person group support, and 6 offered one-on-one telephone support. They noted:

> Community-based peer support programmes are heterogeneous in the format of what they offer and their criteria for who can make use of their support, and mothers with perinatal health difficulties have diverse needs, experiences, and ideas.
>
> (p. 10)

They examined the interactions of context, mechanisms, and outcomes and found 13 context-mechanism-outcome (C-M-O) configurations that explained the positive effects of peer support (McLeish et al., 2023). Empathetic listening, acceptance, affirmation, and normalization led to positive results. Peers shared ideas about self-care, coping, and services, and there were meaningful relationships between mothers and volunteers. Peers sharing their own experiences were especially helpful because they normalized mothers' experiences that seemed abnormal to them. Peer advice sometimes contradicted healthcare providers' advice, but mothers saw peer advice as more realistic. Peer support did not work when mothers did not feel validated, when they criticized themselves in comparison to the peers, when the relationship with the peer was negative or stressful, when peers were being judgmental or directive, and when mothers were not feeling heard (McLeish et al., 2023). Mothers were also distressed when the relationship ended.

The authors concluded that peer support works in complex ways that are affected by personal and social contexts (McLeish et al., 2023). Peer support should not be considered a lower-cost alternative for professional support, but a complementary intervention. Mothers have different backgrounds and needs. They also have different ideas about peer support and whether it will be helpful. Once mothers decide to use peer support, contextual factors, such as the nature of support provided, determine whether it will be a positive or negative experience.

A program from rural Pakistan, in a lower-income rural area north of the Punjab province, invited mothers who had a PHQ-9 score of 10 or higher to participate in a program using *chilla* (LeMasters et al., 2020). *Chilla* is a traditional practice defined as a 40-day confinement after birth where women return to their own mothers' homes and are fed fortifying foods, exempted from housework, and received additional support. They noted that the postpartum depression rate in rural Pakistan was 31%, which is higher than it is in other low- to middle-income countries (LMIC). The women were assessed at 3, 6, 12, 24, and 36 months. Eight hundred and twenty-three mothers completed all the assessments, out of 1,154 who started in the study. Most of the women participated in *chilla* (89%), and 80% were satisfied with it. The women who participated were more educated, had more baseline support, and had lower baseline depression. Mothers with lower depression scores had more positive experiences.

The largest effect was for those with prenatal depression (LeMasters et al., 2020). The authors found that *chilla* was related to perceived social support and embodied the six structures of cultures that prevent postpartum depression outlined by Stern and Kruckman's (1983) classic article, which was described in Volume 1. The authors concluded that *chilla* was a culturally appropriate treatment for maternal mental illness.

Healthcare Provider Support

In addition to peers, healthcare providers can also support new mothers. In a study of 2,064 women, half were assigned to an intervention of flexible care provided by midwives, and the other half were assigned to standard care. At 4 months postpartum, women in the flexible-care group had significantly better mental health than women in the standard-care group. The authors concluded that midwife-led, flexible, tailored-to-individual-needs care significantly improved new mothers' mental health and reduced the risk of postpartum depression (MacArthur et al., 2002).

Pediatric and Adult Primary Care

Pediatric primary care is a key location for providing new-mother support. A review of the literature examined the effects of 18 programs that treated depression in mothers of infants (Olin et al., 2016). Twelve of the 18 programs were pediatric primary care. They all used screening tools and psychosocial risk assessments–guided care. Common strategies were brief counseling, which included motivating mothers to seek help, engaging social support, and facilitating referrals.

Making referrals was the most common strategy in pediatric (83%) and adult primary care (67%) (Olin et al., 2016). Inability to bill for services was a barrier to care, even though their interventions reduced rates of postpartum depression. The authors noted that while managing postpartum depression in a pediatric practice is feasible, more outcome data are needed. The studies describing efficacy were more clinically focused and were often not randomized, nor did they confirm diagnoses after an initial positive screen. However, these studies suggest that treatment could work in this setting and is an avenue worth pursuing.

How Support Is Provided

Community support does not necessarily need to be delivered in person. This is a cost and efficiency issue. None of the studies (to date) used Zoom, but that could also be a viable way to support mothers who have access to a computer, especially when there are no providers in their area. The COVID-19 pandemic opened many alternative ways of offering support, but they were not equally effective. This section describes studies on telephone and digital support.

Telephone Support

A review of six studies compared telephone to in-person peer support as an intervention for postpartum depression (Leger & Letourneau, 2015). Telephone support was as effective as in-person support, with time and cost being two large advantages. The barriers they identified included difficulties making first contact with mothers, the time commitment to provide continuous support, and ethnic and cultural differences. Some of the studies included peers who were trained but had never had postpartum depression so could not provide empathetic support. The authors speculated that lack of empathetic support could explain their null effects.

Telephone support was helpful in preventing postpartum depression in a Canadian study (Dennis et al., 2009). An online screening system identified 701 women as being at high-risk for depression. Mothers were randomized into standard care or telephone support. The supporter was another mother who had recovered from postpartum depression. Peers were matched to the mothers based on ethnicity and area where they lived. Volunteers initiated contact 48 to 72 hours after randomization and were asked to contact mothers at least 4 times, and then as many as they deemed necessary. Women received, on average, 8 contacts. The retention rate among the volunteers was high, suggesting that volunteers also found it rewarding. At 12 and 24 weeks postpartum, a research nurse blinded to treatment conditions followed up by telephone. At 12 weeks, incidence of depression was 14% in the intervention group, and 25% in the control group. Over 80% of women in the intervention group were satisfied with it and would recommend it to a friend. The authors concluded that telephone support was an accessible intervention and effective for mothers from diverse cultures.

A randomized trial from Pittsburgh, US included 628 women who screened positive for depression (EPDS >10) with a follow-up clinical interview (Wisner et al., 2017). Women were randomized to intervention (telephone-delivered depression care management) or control (enhanced usual care) conditions. Enhanced usual care was depression education at a home visit, time to ask questions from a knowledgeable clinician, and they were encouraged to contact their healthcare providers. Depression care management (DCM) was a home visit from a master's-level clinician who became their care manager. Initial calls were 15 to 20 minutes, with 10-minute subsequent calls. Educational materials were provided. The goal of DCM was patient self-management, ongoing education, and supporting shared decision-making, including decisions about medication used during breastfeeding, monitoring symptoms, providing feedback on progress, facilitating access to mental health services, encouraging links to community services, and supporting primary care and mental health practitioners through consultations with perinatal mental health specialists. Case managers reviewed cases weekly. At 6 months, the case manager considered whether mothers had made sufficient progress to discontinue the calls.

Mothers were assessed at 3, 6, and 12 months (Wisner et al., 2017). Depression decreased by greater than 50% for both groups, and the groups did not differ from each other. A subgroup of child sexual abuse survivors responded more favorably to depression care management. They found that regular telephone availability of a clinician was particularly therapeutic.

Another review found that proactive telephone support, where providers initiated the contact, helped with at least four areas related to maternal/child health: preventing smoking relapse, preventing low birthweight, increasing breastfeeding duration and exclusivity, and decreasing the risk of postpartum depression (Dennis & Kingston, 2008). The authors indicated that telephone support, delivered by professionals or peers, is a flexible, efficient, cost-effective, and accessible form of healthcare. Telephone support can be the primary intervention, or it can be a component of larger program.

Postpartum Support International has recently launched a helpline for mothers in the United States. (Mothers in other countries could also probably call but might need to use a different telephone number.) This helpline is staffed 24/7 by trained mental health providers and is an amazing way for mothers to get help when they need it.

1-800-944-4773
Text in English: 800-944-4773
Text en Español: 971-203-7773

Digital Support

Digital support is another cost-effective option for supporting new mothers. A couple of programs have tried online peer support. A content analysis of 512 posted online in a postpartum depression forum revealed that mothers gave and received emotional and instrumental support to each other via this forum (Evans et al., 2012). Emotional support was the most common type. However, not all sites are equally helpful. The researchers recommended that clinicians vet sites before referring mothers to them to ensure that mothers were receiving sound information and that comments were moderated and stayed respectful.

Self-help can also be delivered digitally, where mothers complete a treatment protocol at home with books, DVDs, and websites. For example, a mother may use a book or teaching videos to learn cognitive-behavioral therapy. A meta-analysis of 9 studies examined self-help interventions for postpartum depression (Lin et al., 2018). Six studies found that depressive symptoms decreased after the intervention. The meta-analysis concluded that self-help techniques were an effective way to treat postpartum depression. Depressive symptoms continued to decline from baseline to posttreatment and subsequent follow-up. These changes were greater than in control groups.

A randomized trial from Turkey assigned 62 mothers to use a mobile app that provided postpartum support, which was designed to lower mothers' depression and anxiety levels. They were compared with 62 mothers in the control group who received usual care (Kocak et al., 2021). Most of the mothers in the app group exclusively breastfed and felt more efficient breastfeeding. However, while the depression symptoms were lower in the app group, the app alone did not decrease depression and anxiety symptoms during the 6-week trial. However, it did help mothers access reliable information.

China has 19 apps related to postpartum depression that are available via three platforms (iOS, android, and WeChat) (Li et al., 2020). A review coded the content and functionality of the apps and used the Mobile App Rating Scale (MARS) to assess the app on engagement, functionality, aesthetics, and information. Expert reviewers found that mothers had low adherence with apps and most apps were rated poorly. The app content was monotonous and unlikely to keep the user's interest. In addition, the only metric data developers collected was number of downloads, with follow-up to assess engagement. Of the 19 apps they reviewed, only Overcome Postpartum Anxiety and Depression met all five of their criteria. Despite expansion of the number of apps available for postpartum depression in the Chinese market, they found significant problems and low levels of adherence to clinical practice–based guidelines.

Clinical Takeaways

- In designing your program, realistically consider the types of community support you can provide. There may already be a program in your community that you can partner with.
- Telephone support may allow you to reach more mothers and provide more cost-effective care.
- One advantage of using healthcare providers as supporters is that you can bill insurance for their services.
- If you want to use peer support, I recommend that you pay your peer supporters, if at all possible, so that they can continue to participate and meet the financial needs of their families.

15 Home Visiting, Education, and Infant Massage

Support for new mothers can also take place at home, with home visits provided by peers or professionals. Education is often a part of new mother support. And many community programs also offer infant massage as a modality to help mothers connect with their infants and be more responsive to their cues. It can also help prevent or treat depression.

KEY FINDINGS

- Community support programs often offer home visiting, education, and infant massage.
- Home visiting and infant massage can lower women's risk for depression. Home visiting can prevent depression even when mothers' mental health is not the primary purpose for the visit.
- Education alone does not prevent depression (i.e., simply telling people about depression will not necessarily prevent it). However, mothers may find resources more quickly if they have had some education about it.
- Infant massage releases oxytocin in both mother and baby through the oxytocin receptors on the baby's skin and the palms of mothers' hands. Oxytocin downregulates the stress response, which lowers mothers' risk for depression.

Home Visiting

Home visiting is the most labor-intensive and costly form of new mother support. Home visits are provided by either healthcare providers or trained volunteers. It is standard practice in many countries around the world, but not in the United States. That being said, individual US communities have pooled resources so they could provide this type of support.

Many providers believe that home visiting is uniquely effective. Home visitors see mothers *in situ* and therefore can more accurately evaluate their needs. The setting is also relaxed so that mothers may express concerns that they might not share in a busy clinic. Home visiting has been used to prevent child abuse (Eckenrode et al., 2010), lower the risk of postpartum depression (Milani et al., 2017), and increase breastfeeding rates (Edwards et al., 2013). The type of services offered, and the quality of the support, vary widely between programs, however. Poor conceptualization or implementation of a home visiting program might result null or negative findings. And sometimes what works is not what you would expect. Here is an example.

DOI: 10.4324/9781003405092-18

An Iranian study of 276 postpartum women randomized them into either home-visiting or usual-care conditions (Milani et al., 2017). Mothers completed the EPDS before delivery and at 60 days postpartum. Mothers who were depressed at Time 1 were excluded. The results were impressive. The rate of depression in the home-visiting group was 8% vs. 19% in the control group. Consistent with previous findings, mothers who were not exclusively breastfeeding were 2.25 times more likely to be depressed.

The surprise is that intervention had any impact on mothers' mental health since the program did not address it at all (Milani et al., 2017). The home visitors were trained midwives who interviewed mothers and completed checklists about the mothers' physical health and nutrition "based on her socioeconomic status." Mothers received two 45-minute visits. They did not provide mental health support, but simply *being there* seemed to offer support. That is consistent with a meta-analysis on randomized controlled trials (RCTs) that sought to prevent postpartum depression. In this analysis, type of intervention was not related to reducing depressive symptoms or preventing them. They concluded that "non-specific social contact and support was sufficient for reducing risk for depression" (p. 1,215) (Sockol et al., 2013).

A review considered whether US state-level interventions on postpartum depression were effective (Rowan et al., 2015). They identified 13 states that had enacted one or more peripartum mental health practices, including patient education materials, mandated depression screening, mandated task forces, and public awareness campaigns. Available evidence suggests most of the interventions had little impact. However, home visits with a mental health component were effective for postpartum depression.

A study from South Africa found that home visiting improved mother–infant interaction but did not decrease depression (Cooper, 2002). In this study, 32 women were randomly assigned to receive home visits by trained community volunteers or usual care. The home visitors provided emotional support and taught mothers to be more responsive to their babies using items from the Neonatal Behavioral Assessment Scale. This intervention had no significant impact on maternal mood (although it was better for mothers in the intervention group). But it was significantly associated with mothers being more positive with their babies.

Skin-to-skin contact immediately after birth, and for the first month postpartum, can also prevent depression (Bigelow et al., 2012). This intervention was administered by home visitors, and mothers recorded their times. With skin-to-skin contact, mothers hold their babies between their breasts, with the infants wearing only their diapers, with a blanket on their backs. Mothers can also wear something around their shoulders. Thirty women were randomized to the skin-to-skin group, and 60 mothers were in the control group. Mothers in the intervention group held their babies skin-to-skin approximately 5 hours a day during the first week, and 2 hours a day until the end of the first month. The mothers in the skin-to-skin group had lower depression scores at the end of the first week, likely due to increased oxytocin. They also had lower salivary cortisol during the first month. After week 1, the effects diminished, with no differences between the groups at 2 and 3 months. Surprisingly, this study did not control for breastfeeding, which is a significant potential confound, because breastfeeding (with milk ejection) increases oxytocin and lowers cortisol (Heinrichs et al., 2001). So the question remains, Did the skin-to-skin contact lower cortisol above and beyond skin-to-skin contact that is a natural part of breastfeeding? There is no way to answer that question with this study design.

Another study used teams of nurses and peer community health workers, with a sample of 613 low-income, Medicaid-eligible American women (Del Castillo & Wright, 2009). Women were randomized to either usual-care or nurse/community-health-worker conditions. The nurses made two prenatal visits, one post-delivery, and at least two additional visits in the first year.

The community health workers provided relationship-based support via phone and face-to-face contacts (Del Castillo & Wright, 2009). They saw mothers every other week during pregnancy, and every week for the first month postpartum. At 2 to 6 months, contact dropped to every other week, and after 6 months, they evaluated the situation. If needed, they continued to see the mothers either every other week or once a month. Mothers in the intervention received, on average, 24 visits, compared with 8.5 visits in the usual-care group. The results indicated that the women who received support from the nurse/community health worker teams had significantly lower depressive symptoms. This was especially true for women who had low resources and high stress. There were no differences between the groups for social support or self-esteem.

Education

Education is a key component of many community-based programs that aim to reduce the risk of depression and help mothers have more positive interactions with their babies. However, many programs are poorly done, with communities relying solely on education for their intervention (such as including a handout in the discharge packet). It seems like magical thinking to believe that simply *telling* someone about postpartum depression makes them less susceptible. It might help mothers locate resources if they become depressed, or they may seek treatment sooner, but it does not prevent it. Studies have consistently found that education alone is ineffective. However, it can be a useful adjunct with other types of support.

Many education interventions involve only one session. For example, a US study examined an education intervention for new mothers at three time points (McCarter-Spaulding & Shea, 2016). One hundred twenty mothers and their partners (if present) received a handout on depression at discharge, and its contents were discussed for 5 to 20 minutes. These mothers were compared to those who received usual care. There was no significant difference in depression rates at any of the three screening points (6 weeks, 3 and 6 months).

A study from the Netherlands randomized 138 women and 96 partners into either intervention or wait-list conditions. The intervention group received a booklet and video, a home visit, and a telephone call at 4 weeks (Missler et al., 2020). Parents were educated during pregnancy about caring for themselves while caring for their infants, infant crying patterns, and feeding and sleep arrangements. Postpartum stress was the primary outcome. Secondary outcomes were postpartum depression and anxiety. There was no difference between the intervention and wait-list groups on postpartum stress, anxiety, or depression, as both groups were highly stressed. In addition, the education program did not impact caregiving. Interestingly, mothers in the intervention group reported *more* parenting problems than the control group, but they liked the educational booklet.

Similarly, a study from Denmark found that a short antenatal education program for first-time mothers did not prevent postpartum depression (Maimburg & Vaeth, 2015).

Six hundred and three pregnant women participated in the Ready for Child program, and 590 mothers received standard care. The Ready for Child program was a 9-hour class that prepared women for labor and discussed issues related to infant care and postpartum adjustment, including postpartum depression. They found that lack of breastfeeding increased the risk for postpartum depression, but that antenatal education program did not lower women's risk.

Another study combined education and motivational interviewing to encourage depressed mothers to contact community resources (Fernandez y Garcia et al., 2015). In this sample from California, 104 mothers of children 0 to 12 months old were randomized to either control or Motivating Our Mothers (MOMS) conditions. Mothers in both groups received a list of resources. The MOMS intervention included a pamphlet and a structured 5-minute interview meant to motivate them to access free parenting and depression resources. The second part was a 15-minute semi-structured telephone call that reviewed the same content 2 days later. The primary outcome was whether depressed mothers reached out for help. At the end of the program, 74% of intervention mothers, and 54% in the control group, accessed depression and parenting assistance.

Similarly, a study of 540 predominantly White affluent mothers participated in a two-step intervention that educated them on modifiable risk factors for depression, improved their level of social support, and enhanced their overall management skills (Howell et al., 2014). Mothers were randomized into the treatment or control (usual care) conditions. Researchers assessed depression at 3 weeks, 3 months, and 6 months postpartum, and there was no difference between the groups, mainly because depression was low at all time periods in both groups, ranging from 3% to 6%.

Infant Massage

Infant massage is a surprising entry into the arsenal of community-based treatments. I've included it in this section because it is often part of community-based programs. From a physiological standpoint, infant massage makes sense as an intervention. All humans have oxytocin receptors on the palms of their hands. Massage increases oxytocin in mothers and infants, which suppresses stress, which lowers mothers' risk for depression. Massage is also an effective way for mothers and babies to connect, particularly if mothers had difficult births or were disengaging from their babies. I did not include massage in the previous edition because most of the research was quite old. However, we now have some new studies, and I thought it was important to provide an update.

Two older studies from the UK found that infant massage helped with depression and improved mother–infant interactions. The first was a small pilot study with 12 mothers in the massage group and 13 in the control group (Glover et al., 2002). All the mothers had scored over 13 on the EPDS. By the end of the study, depressive symptoms improved for both groups, but more for the mothers in the massage group than the control group. Mothers' interactions with their babies also improved. Massage relaxed mother and baby, increased maternal confidence, increased maternal understanding of their babies' cues, and released oxytocin, which promoted bonding.

The second study by this same group assigned 34 depressed mothers to infant-massage or support-group conditions (Onozawa et al., 2001). There were five weekly sessions. The EPDS scores fell in both groups by the end of 5 weeks, with a larger effect in the infant-massage group. There was also significant improvement in mother–infant interaction in the massage group compared to the support group.

More recently, a randomized trial with 138 mothers receiving treatment for substance use, compared parent education, parent education with infant massage, and a control group on parenting stress, depression, self-esteem, mother–infant attachment, and mother–infant interaction after 5 weeks (Porter et al., 2015). The control group received usual care. The infant massage program taught mothers to apply gentle strokes and kneading while singing or talking with their infants. The materials were translated into both Spanish and Creole to reflect the large Hispanic and Haitian communities in South Florida. Both intervention groups had significantly decreased stress and depression compared to controls at 12 weeks, with a "slightly greater" change for the massage/education group. But there were no differences in self-esteem, attachment, or interaction. In addition, the infant massage/education group showed significant improvement in stress over time. The mothers' lowered stress was also reflected in measures of their waist-to-hip ratio, with higher abdominal weight being a physical manifestation of chronic stress—and a potential risk factor for later health problems. The other groups did not have this sustained effect.

The authors concluded that infant massage added value to the education program because it decreased stress and depression above and beyond an educational program (Porter et al., 2015). They noted that birth of an infant exposed to substances in utero is both a crisis and an opportunity for recovery for mothers. The researchers described their education/massage intervention as "low-input, high-impact" because it improved mothers' physical and mental health in a particularly high-risk group.

The effect of infant massage appears quickly. Seventy mothers of preterm infants from Iran were assessed for anxiety 24 hours before their infants were due to be discharged (Afand et al., 2016). They were then randomized to either massage or control conditions. Mothers in the massage group were given 8 minutes of instruction on infant massage, which they learned by massaging their infants with an instructor. All 70 mothers were reassessed on the day of discharge. Anxiety dropped for both groups once infants were discharged, but it was significantly lower for mothers who were instructed in infant massage.

Another Iranian study used a quasi-experimental design to examine the effects of infant massage on 120 mothers with babies in the NICU (Rahmatnezhad et al., 2018). The intervention group received 3 days of midwife-led instruction on infant massage. The control group (usual care) had no improvement between Time 1 (admission) and Time 2 (discharge) on awareness, perceived stress, and breastfeeding self-efficacy, while the intervention group significantly improved in all three.

Although these results are positive, there were some significant methodological issues that damper my enthusiasm for this study. The main concern was the study design. The researchers selected and assessed the control group first, before they recruited the intervention group, and then used a quasi-experimental design. Normally, a quasi-experimental design is used when there are pre-existing groups and randomization would be unethical (e.g., groups of children who were either abused or non-abused, mothers who breastfed or who did not). In this case, however, randomization was possible as it was a convenience sample drawn from a local NICU; mothers could have been assigned to either group. The authors may have introduced bias into their findings by not randomizing their sample. Randomization generally lowers bias by controlling for inadvertent or unconscious selection of people into groups. I am pleased to see these results, and they are consistent with other studies, but this would be a poor study to base policy on when there are others with sounder methodologies.

A review of 19 articles on postpartum depression examined studies related to the mother–infant relationship (Lindensmith, 2018). The author concluded that infant massage had a positive impact on the mother–infant relationship. The results for education and psychotherapy were mixed; some studies found that these interventions helped, while others did not. Most of the 19 studies were on psychotherapy, but many of the studies had small sample sizes. The results of the larger studies were mixed. (In fairness, the primary goal of psychotherapy was to improve mothers' mental health, not the mother–infant relationship.) The education intervention was mother–infant coaching, which can be very effective. It is more interactive than the straight education programs I described in the previous section.

Infant massage was included as an intervention in 4 studies (including 1 case study), with 1 having null results (cited previously in this section) (Lindensmith, 2018). Of the 5 studies she reviewed on infant massage, 3 plus the case study had positive results. While the author considered infant massage a superior intervention, a close reading of findings reveals that the results are mixed. It seems safe to say that all three interventions appear to be effective most of the time.

Oxytocin facilitates mother–infant bonding and is released in mother and baby during massage and skin-to-skin contact. As such, researchers have hypothesized that infant massage might benefit mothers who have disordered bonding with their infants. A study of 37 mother–infant dyads from Egypt examined mother and infant salivary oxytocin pre- and post-infant massage (Moussa et al., 2021). Forty-nine percent of the dyads had disordered bonding as determined by their scores on the Postpartum Bonding Questionnaire. The questionnaire measured mothers' feelings about their infants. The authors said surprisingly little about the content of this scale or what a high score meant. Only that it was problematic. For dyads with normal bonding, oxytocin increased post massage in both mothers and infants. In contrast, *massage did not increase oxytocin in either mothers or babies who had disordered bonding*. These findings are concerning because an intervention that might have been helpful for these mothers was not. And it is unclear why. I hope this finding leads to more research.

Another unique finding was the sex difference in oxytocin response (Moussa et al., 2021). The male infants' pre-massage oxytocin levels were significantly higher than in female infants. However, for males in the normal bonding group, oxytocin decreased post-massage, but it increased in females. The authors noted that oxytocin receptor activity is usually higher in females. These findings are also of interest and are consistent with studies I described in Volume I, where males were more likely to have sensitive temperaments and sleep disorders. It is unclear how those findings fit together, but they are in the same direction so would be worth exploring in future studies.

Summary

Community-based social support shows promise in helping women make a smooth transition to motherhood. To be most effective, community-based programs must take place alongside more traditional, individually focused interventions for depression. Moreover, we need research that demonstrates the effectiveness of these programs in preventing or ameliorating postpartum depression.

Clinical Takeaways

- Home visiting can help new mothers adjust to their new role. However, it can be costly to implement so may be out of reach when just starting a program. Telephone support, described in the previous section, may be a more cost-effective alternative.
- Simply adding educational materials to discharge packets, or even discussing them with new families, does not prevent depression. Psychoeducation can be an important part of treatment, but it is not a treatment by itself.
- Infant massage can be a great way for mothers and infants to reconnect, especially after a difficult birth. It also downregulates the stress response that underlies depression so lowers risk.

Section IV
Psychotherapy

16 Cognitive-Behavioral Therapy

Psychotherapy is another way mothers can increase support as they navigate new motherhood. In clinical trials, psychotherapy was as effective as medications in treating depression, with lower rates of relapse (Claridge, 2014; Rupke et al., 2006). A meta-analysis of 24 studies found a large effect size of psychotherapy for one group in particular: perinatal women (Claridge, 2014). The effect sizes were the same for pregnancy and postpartum, reducing depression in both time periods. Chapters 16 and 17 examine cognitive-behavioral therapy and interpersonal psychotherapy for postpartum depression. Both are considered frontline treatments for depression in new mothers and treat anxiety and PTSD.

KEY FINDINGS

- CBT is an effective form of psychotherapy for new mothers. It helps with depression, anxiety, and PTSD, with results comparable to medications.
- Mindfulness has been added to cognitive therapy with good results. This type of therapy includes mindful techniques, such as breath awareness, mindful movement, and body awareness.
- Self-compassion is a component of mindfulness that encompasses self-kindness. This creates resilience when mothers encounter difficult situations.
- Cognitive therapy also addresses negative thought patterns that increase inflammation. Part of its therapeutic effect is its physiological downregulation of the stress system by changing negative ways of looking at the world.

In numerous randomized trials, cognitive-behavioral therapy (CBT) was as effective as medications and changed the brain in the same way. CBT treats depression, anxiety, chronic pain, obsessive-compulsive disorder, and PTSD (Marchesi, 2008; Marchesi et al., 2016; Rupke et al., 2006; Speisman et al., 2011). Patients who received cognitive therapy were less likely to relapse and drop out of treatment than those who received medications alone.

Cognitive therapy is based on the premise that distortions in thinking cause depression. It teaches patients to recognize and counter these distorted thoughts (Rupke et al., 2006). The core deficit is called the negative cognitive triad: individuals' negative views of themselves, their worlds, and their future (O'Hara & Engeldinger, 2018). This leads to negative schemas (ways of looking at the world) that possibly developed in early life and become filters for current experience or thought. When experiencing stressors or loss, people with a negative or pessimistic worldview process those events in a way that leads

DOI: 10.4324/9781003405092-20

to depression (blaming themselves for the event, thinking it will never change, and that it will affect every area of their lives).

Cognitive therapy is *not* simply learning to think "happy" thoughts or to ignore or minimize reality. Instead, the goal is to help patients identify distorted beliefs and replace them with rational ones. Changing thinking changes the brain (Barsaglini et al., 2014). Cognitive therapy typically lasts 10 to 20 sessions over 12 to 16 weeks. Early sessions focus on making clients more behaviorally active. Later sessions address dysfunctional beliefs. Sessions include problem-solving, goal-setting, and role-playing (O'Hara & Engeldinger, 2018).

When used for postpartum depression, CBT focuses on the mother's relationship with her infant and includes practicing with the therapist to help mothers advocate for what they need in their new role. The behavioral aspect helps clients identify specific problems that are maintaining their depression. Interventions include assignments that increase mastery and pleasure, problem-solving, breaking down large goals into smaller parts, and minimizing avoidance as a strategy to cope with difficult problems.

A study from Australia compared standard care, group cognitive therapy, or individual counseling for women with postpartum depression. After 12 weeks, both types of psychological treatment were superior to standard care, and the researchers concluded that individual counseling was as effective as group cognitive therapy (Milgrom et al., 2005). A more recent study randomized 45 women with postpartum major depression to cognitive-behavioral therapy, sertraline, or a combination of both (Milgrom et al., 2015). The mothers were assessed at 12 and 24 weeks. Depression and anxiety were reduced in all three groups, but cognitive-behavioral therapy as a monotreatment was more effective than the other two conditions. Mothers in the CBT monotherapy group had the most rapid initial gains when they started treatment. There was no detectable advantage to adding medication to CBT.

Researchers added cognitive therapy to medications to treat moderate to severe postpartum depression in another study (Misri et al., 2004). Depressed, anxious mothers were assigned to receive paroxetine alone, or paroxetine with group cognitive therapy. Mothers in both groups improved after treatment, and there was no significant difference between the groups. The authors concluded that cognitive therapy did not add to medications, perhaps because the medications were already addressing the symptoms.

A small trial of 23 mothers with postpartum depression tested whether reducing depressive symptoms lowered parenting stress (Misri et al., 2006). Mothers were randomized to receive either medication or cognitive-behavioral therapy. All the mothers had clinically significant levels of parenting stress before treatment. At the end of the study, both cognitive therapy and medication monotherapy decreased maternal stress. Rather than targeting stress directly, both treatments lowered postpartum depression, which also lowered parenting stress.

A study from Korea randomly assigned 27 pregnant women with depression to either a cognitive-behavioral therapy (CBT) or a control condition (Cho et al., 2008). CBT happened during pregnancy and consisted of 9 bi-weekly, one-on-one, 1-hour sessions. The components included educating patients about depression, scheduling pleasant events, and changing negative thoughts to positive ones. Regarding marital relationships, the intervention promoted understanding of their spouses. In the control group, patients were educated about depression in one prenatal session. The authors found that CBT administered during pregnancy prevented postpartum depression, and it improved marital satisfaction. The intervention used standard CBT techniques but focused on behavioral techniques to improve marital relationships.

Cognitive therapy did not prevent depression in mothers of very preterm babies (Hagan et al., 2004). In this study, 101 mothers of babies of very preterm infants received 6 sessions of cognitive therapy. They were compared with 98 mothers who received standard care. Thirty seven percent of the mothers were depressed. There were no differences in onset or duration of depression between the two groups. Mothers of very preterm infants had high rates of stress and depression, and a 6-week intervention was not sufficient to prevent depression in this group.

A review of 18 studies found that cognitive-behavioral therapy was effective for treating perinatal anxiety disorders, including obsessive-compulsive disorder, panic disorder, and specific phobias (Marchesi et al., 2016). The authors recommended cognitive therapy as a frontline treatment because of its safety and efficacy. Selective-serotonin reuptake inhibitors (SSRIs) are effective treatments during pregnancy and increase the risk of prematurity and low birthweight. In late pregnancy, SSRI use has been associated with poor neonatal adaptation and persistent pulmonary hypertension (although this complication is rare). See Chapter 21 for more details.

CBT can even be delivered by peers. Seventy-three mothers in Ontario, Canada, were randomized into experimental or wait-list conditions (Amani et al., 2022). All had scores of 10 or greater on the EPDS. The peers were trained and supervised by the study authors. The intervention was 9 sessions, 2 hours each. The first hour was devoted to core skills, such as cognitive restructuring, behavioral activation, relaxation, and goal-setting. The second hour was unstructured and included discussion about relevant issues, such as sleep and social support. The outcomes were assessed at 6 months postpartum. The peers provided the CBT for postpartum depression and anxiety, which significantly improved in the treatment group compared to the wait-list group. Prior to treatment, mothers believed that they had impaired bonding, that their babies were rejecting them, and they were angry about it. These negative beliefs decreased during CBT. Commenting on this article, O'Hara (2022) noted that what set this study apart from other "peer" studies was that it used a validated psychological intervention. This study also suggests that common mental health problems can be addressed by people without formal mental health training, which, as Amani et al. suggest, makes the intervention scalable.

A study from Quebec raised one limitation to cognitive-behavioral therapy. In their study of CBT as a treatment for PTSD, Belleville and colleagues (2011) assessed 55 patients with PTSD before treatment, and 6 months after. They found that many of the sleep parameters improved after treatment, but these improvements were not maintained after 6 months. Of the people who had sleep problems at baseline, 70% still had significant sleep problems after treatment. Sleep problems were associated with more depression, anxiety, and poorer health. Although cognitive therapy does improve sleep, there were still residual sleep difficulties, and this may be a particular issue for perinatal women with PTSD.

Mindfulness-Based Cognitive Therapy

A recent variant of cognitive therapy incorporates mindfulness and is known as mindfulness-based cognitive therapy (MBCT). It contains the same elements as traditional cognitive therapy but also incorporates practices of mindfulness. Mindfulness is a 2,500-year-old practice recently incorporated into Western medicine to reduce stress in adults (Bluth & Blanton, 2014). Mindfulness is a state of consciousness that brings awareness and attention to someone's immediate experience. It is both an outcome and a process. It teaches participants to hold negative thoughts in awareness and accept them with a non-judgmental and compassionate attitude.

Mindfulness is a secular application of a technique originally derived from Buddhism. It involves paying attention to everyday experiences that people usually ignore: the taste of coffee, the sensation of walking down the stairs, the sound of rain on the roof, the texture and taste of a raisin. The theory behind MBCT is that life stress leads to dysphoria, which leads to negative thinking and negative affect, which leads to depression. MBCT interrupts this cycle and decreases emotional reactivity. It is effective because it regulates intensity of an emotional response and includes reappraisal. Cognitive control is the ability to sustain attention in the face of distracting information. These mechanisms are part of a protocol for a randomized trial designed to understand why MBCT would be effective for pregnant depressed women (Seghete et al., 2020). Practicing mindfulness has two key components:

- Being *aware* in the present moment.
- *Accepting* thoughts and feelings without judging them.

Clients are asked to spend daily time dedicated to practicing mindful techniques, such as breath awareness, mindful movement (e.g., gentle yoga), and body awareness. When going through difficulties, mindfulness neither represses suffering nor allows it to overwhelm them. It acknowledges it but also recognizes that the situation is temporary (Mahurin-Smith & Beck, 2022). In a meta-analysis of 41 trials involving 2,993 participants, MBCT lowered anxiety, depression, and pain (Goyal et al., 2014).

Self-Compassion

Self-compassion is a component of mindfulness and encompasses self-kindness. It is frequently combined with mindfulness in intervention studies. Self-compassion recognizes that we are part of common humanity and can have balanced awareness of our emotional experiences (Bluth & Blanton, 2014). It also includes self-kindness over self-judgment, which creates resilience (Mahurin-Smith & Beck, 2022). It is not the same as self-esteem.

A retrospective survey of 318 women with self-reported breastfeeding problems found that higher self-compassion was associated with significantly less postpartum depression and anxiety (Mahurin-Smith & Beck, 2022). The researchers measured severity of the breastfeeding problems, the importance of breastfeeding to the mothers, and postpartum depression and anxiety. Mothers completed the Self-Compassion Scale. Mothers with high self-compassion might say things like, "Many other mothers have breastfeeding problems." They found that each unit increase on the Self-Compassion Scale was associated with a 41% decrease in postpartum depression or anxiety.

While these findings are promising, there is a strong limitation that must be considered: directionality of the findings (Mahurin-Smith & Beck, 2022). The findings from this study are retrospective. Did self-compassion precede depression or anxiety, or did anxiety or depression influence mothers' ability to perceive events in a self-compassionate way? The authors also recognized this limitation. However, the findings raise another interesting issue: is it possible to teach self-compassion to help new mothers navigate postpartum?

A Chinese study demonstrated that teaching self-compassion was feasible. Researchers adapted an English-language version of a Mindfulness-Based Self-Compassion Program (Guo et al., 2020). It was a 6-week program with 10 hours of training over 36 episodes (6/week). Each lasted 15 minutes. The study included 144 women in the treatment group and 140 in the control group. Mothers were included if they were in the second or third trimester of pregnancy and had an EPDS score of 9 or more. They also needed Internet access and could speak Chinese. At 3 months, the EPDS scores dropped below 9 for the intervention group, with a mild decrease between 3 and 12 months. In contrast, there was no change in EPDS scores for the control group. Both groups improved in parenting stress over the 12 months, but the intervention group showed more improvement. Maternal warmth also improved. The dropout rate was low, and the mothers reported that it was a positive experience.

Effectiveness Studies

A pilot study from South Australia included 10 pregnant women in the treatment group, and 9 in the control group (Dunn et al., 2012). The treatment involved an 8-week program. The researchers found that 75% of the mothers in the treatment group experienced a decrease in stress symptoms at 6 weeks postpartum, but there was little change for mothers in the control group. Fifty percent of mothers in the mindfulness group experienced a positive change in their depression scores on the EPDS.

A study of 30 mothers had similar findings with an 8-week mindfulness-based cognitive therapy program (Shulman et al., 2018). The mothers were recruited from a maternal mental health clinic because their depression did not remit after being treated with medications. After the 8-week program, they were evaluated at 3 months. There were 14 in the intervention group and 16 in the usual-care group. Most of the effects were not statistically significant but were trending toward it. However, the effect sizes for all three variables were large, suggesting a clinically significant effect of the intervention.

Another small, randomized trial included 26 breastfeeding mothers from Spain (Perez-Blasco et al., 2013). They found that mothers who participated in the mindfulness-based intervention had significantly higher self-efficacy and were higher on self-compassion, acting with awareness, non-judging, and non-reactivity than mothers in the control group. Mothers participated in 8 sessions, where they learned skills, such as mindfulness vs. autopilot, overcoming obstacles, acceptance, emotional debt, self-compassion and compassion, forgiveness, and conscious care. Mothers in the control group received usual care. The authors concluded that a mindfulness-based intervention can improve mothers' well-being and self-efficacy and reduce psychological distress in postpartum women.

A qualitative study of 24 pregnant women with generalized anxiety disorder found that completing the program significantly lowered anxiety, worry, and depression (Goodman et al., 2014). They also had significant increases in self-compassion and mindfulness. The authors concluded that MBCT was an effective, non-pharmacologic treatment for anxiety during pregnancy.

A recent review of meta-analyses found moderate-quality evidence. Cognitive-behavioral therapy not only works but it is also more effective than standard antidepressant treatment for depression in the general population (Haller et al., 2019). They noted that individual studies were often well done, but when their findings were synthesized in meta-analyses, studies may have failed to report findings, which downgraded the evidence.

The Anti-Inflammatory Effects of Cognitive Therapy

Although the evidence is still preliminary, cognitive therapy appears to have an anti-inflammatory effect (Kiecolt-Glaser et al., 2015). To understand this, it is helpful to examine the literature on the health effects of hostility. Hostility is of interest because it is a particular worldview that CBT can address. People high in hostility tend to attribute negative motives to others, have difficulty trusting others and establishing close relationships. Hostility also specifically raises inflammation. In one study, hostility was associated with higher levels of circulating proinflammatory cytokines (IL-1α, IL-1β, and IL-8) in 44 healthy, non-smoking, premenopausal women. The combination of depression and hostility led to the highest levels of IL-1β, IL-8, and TNF-α (Suarez et al., 2004). There was a dose-response effect: the more severe the depression and hostility, the greater the production of cytokines.

In another study, Suarez (2006) studied 135 healthy patients (75 men, 60 women) with no symptoms of diabetes. He found that women with higher levels of depression and hostility had higher levels of fasting insulin, glucose, and insulin resistance. These findings were not true for men, and they were independent of other risk factors for metabolic syndrome, including body mass index, age, fasting triglycerides, exercise regularity, or ethnicity. These findings were significant since pre-study glucose levels were in the non-diabetic range. The author noted that inflammation, particularly elevated IL-6 and C-reactive protein, may mediate the relationship between depression and hostility and risk of type 2 diabetes and cardiovascular disease, possibly because they increase insulin resistance.

Kiecolt-Glaser et al. (2005) found that couples who were high in hostility had higher levels of circulating proinflammatory cytokines. As a result, wound healing in high-hostility couples was 60% slower than in low-hostility couples. High-hostility couples had high levels of cytokines circulating systemically, where they were more likely to impair health and increase the risk of age-related diseases.

Cognitive therapy specifically addresses beliefs, such as hostility. Since negative cognitions increase inflammation, reducing occurrence of these beliefs should lower inflammation. That is indeed what Doering and colleagues (2007) found in their study of women after coronary bypass surgery. Clinically depressed women had a higher incidence of in-hospital fevers and infections in the 6 months after surgery, due, in part, to decreases in natural-killer-cell cytotoxicity. An 8-week program of cognitive-behavioral therapy reduced depression, improved natural-killer-cell cytotoxicity, and decreased IL-6 and C-reaction protein. Because the immune system was functioning more effectively, cognitive therapy decreased post-operative infectious diseases.

Cognitive-behavioral therapy lowered C-reactive protein in a sample of 123 older adults with sleep difficulties (Irwin et al., 2014). Sleep improved at 4 months, and C-reactive protein dropped at 16 months. Sleep improvements likely lowered C-reactive protein, but the mechanism is unclear.

Clinical Takeaways

- What we think, and how we frame the world, has a substantial impact on our mental health.
- Cognitive-behavioral therapy treats even major depression and produces changes in the brain comparable to antidepressants.
- It also has no negative impact on fetal development or breastfeeding and is a viable, effective alternative to medications for the treatment of depression.
- Mindfulness is a particularly effective addition to cognitive therapy and improves its outcomes.

17 Interpersonal Psychotherapy

Interpersonal psychotherapy (IPT) is based on attachment theory and the work of psychologist Harry Stack Sullivan. The basic tenet is that depressed people have social problems, such as interpersonal conflicts, problems in role transition, or in managing loss. Disturbances in the key relationships are hypothesized as being responsible for depression (Miniati et al., 2014). Interpersonal psychotherapy addresses four problem areas: role transitions, interpersonal disputes, grief, and interpersonal deficits. It was originally designed as a pragmatic intervention meant to supplement or enhance medication treatment (O'Hara & Engeldinger, 2018). Subsequent research revealed that it worked well on its own and is effective for perinatal women.

KEY FINDINGS

- IPT effectively prevents and treats depression during pregnancy and postpartum.
- It is also effective with high-risk clients who may not be amenable to other treatments.
- IPT is a short-term treatment that can also be administered in group settings and by trained laypeople.
- It is a frontline psychotherapy for perinatal women.

On a client's first visit, one specific problem is identified, and the client and therapist begin work on it. Mothers complete an interpersonal inventory and review information about key relationships, the nature of current communications, and how having a baby has changed those relationships (Grigoriadis & Ravitz, 2007; O'Hara & Engeldinger, 2018). With postpartum women, the goal is to help them with role transitions and navigate changes in roles they have already established. A related goal is to assist women in building support or making better use of support that already exists (Grigoriadis & Ravitz, 2007).

A systematic review of 11 studies examined the efficacy of interpersonal psychotherapy for treating postpartum depression. IPT shortened recovery time for postpartum depression and prolonged clinical remission (Miniati et al., 2014). Miniati et al. (2014) noted that IPT may be even more effective than cognitive therapies for postpartum depression and recommended it as a first-line treatment.

Two review articles also indicated that interpersonal psychotherapy effectively treated postpartum depression. Weissman's (2007) review of 4 clinical trials found that women who received 12 to 16 weeks of interpersonal psychotherapy were significantly less depressed compared to women in the standard-care condition. Weissman also noted that healthcare providers or trained laypeople can deliver interpersonal psychotherapy. Grigoriadis and

DOI: 10.4324/9781003405092-21

Ravitz (2007) concluded that interpersonal psychotherapy effectively treats postpartum depression and that it can be easily integrated into primary care.

Clinical Trials and Perinatal Samples

Interpersonal psychotherapy was used to treat low-income depressed adolescents in five school-based mental health clinics in New York City (Mufson et al., 2004). In this study, 63 teens with depression or dysthymia were randomly assigned to receive 16 weeks of interpersonal psychotherapy or 16 weeks of usual care. Usual care included whatever psychotherapy the teens normally received. The sample was 84% female and 71% Hispanic. At 16 weeks, teens in the IPT group were significantly less depressed, had better social functioning, had greater clinical improvement, and had a larger decrease in clinical severity on the Clinical Global Impressions Scale. The largest treatment effects were for teens who were older and more severely depressed. Although medications are often seen as frontline treatment for depressed teens, they were difficult to access through school clinics. Moreover, minority families were frequently reluctant to accept them. Four teens in the study were prescribed antidepressants, and all had poor compliance. The authors concluded that this school-based IPT program was a viable alternative to medications for depressed low-income adolescents.

Another study compared interpersonal psychotherapy to parent education for 50 low-income pregnant women with major depression (Spinelli, 2003). Women in their sample had several severe risk factors for depression: 47% had a history of childhood abuse (28% sexual abuse, 25% physical abuse, 6% both), and 73% had a history of major depression. In addition, many had chaotic home environments, unstable relationships, or partners involved in criminal activity. At the end of 16 weeks, significantly more women in the treatment group had reduced depressive symptoms by 50% or more on the Hamilton Depression Rating Scale and the Beck Depression Inventory. These authors also recommended IPT as a frontline treatment.

O'Hara and colleagues randomized 162 women with postpartum depression into three groups: IPT, sertraline-clinical management, or pill-placebo clinical management (O'Hara et al., 2019). Treatment lasted 12 weeks. Clinical management included an initial session of 50 minutes, with follow-up sessions that were 20 to 30 minutes. During these sessions, women were asked about symptoms and side effects, encouraged to comply with treatment, assessed in their use of other medications, and clinicians collected their unused pills. Mothers were also asked about the babies and given information about postpartum depression. Mothers could ask questions about their babies, stress, medication, and breastfeeding. (Which sounds a lot like counseling.) Not surprisingly, women in all three conditions improved, with no significant difference between the groups. O'Hara and colleagues used both the PHQ-9 and EPDS to screen for depression, with the Structural Clinical Interview-Depression (SCID) to confirm the diagnosis. Both the placebo and medication conditions were "high contact," 9 sessions over 12 weeks with a psychiatrist. Interestingly, they found a relatively high percentage of women did not comply with treatment, particularly in the sertraline condition.

In a study of 120 women with postpartum major depression (O'Hara et al., 2000), women were assigned to either IPT or wait-list conditions for 12 weeks. The therapists followed a standardized treatment manual. Women who had IPT were significantly less depressed than women in the wait-list group at 4, 8, and 12 weeks after treatment. The rate of recovery from depression was also significantly higher for women in the therapy group, and they scored better on postpartum adjustment and social support. In summary, interpersonal therapy reduced depressive symptoms and improved social adjustment for women with postpartum depression.

Treatment for Partners

Partners can also be treated with IPT in conjunction with mothers. An open-label pilot study of Partner-Assisted IPT included 10 couples for 8 acute-phase sessions and a 6-week follow-up (Brandon et al., 2012). The rationale is that partners derive comfort and security from each other. When one partner is depressed, an extra burden falls on the non-depressed partner to maintain positive interactions. If non-depressed partners do not understand depression, they may respond with withdrawal, anger, and recrimination. The goal is to help partners understand depression and support depressed mothers in their recoveries. Sessions help partners respond in ways that mothers perceive as supportive. At the beginning of the trial, 90% of the women met criteria for depression. At the end of the trial, 89% met criteria for recovery at 6 weeks. The authors concluded that involving partners in treatment was safe, acceptable, and feasible and was a useful component of both treatment and prevention of relapse.

Long-Term Effects

The effects of IPT appear to be long-lasting. In an 18-month follow-up of mothers who received IPT, different trajectories of recovery appeared (Nylen et al., 2010). One-hundred twenty women were randomized to a 12-week IPT treatment group or a wait-list condition. Of the 35 women who recovered in the acute phase, 57% sustained that recovery during follow-up. More than 80% of women who did not recover in the initial phase recovered at some point during follow-up. The authors concluded that IPT led to long-term benefits. Women who did not initially recover during the acute phase might benefit from continued treatment. They also suggested offering maintenance treatment to women who have achieved stable remission.

Another study examined the long-term impact of group IPT at 2 years posttreatment for 50 mothers who had severe postpartum depression (EPDS >13) (Reay et al., 2012). The mothers were randomized to IPT or usual-care conditions. The IPT group received two individual sessions, eight 2-hour group sessions, and a 2-hour partners' evening. Women who participated in group IPT improved more rapidly, were significantly less likely to develop persistent depressive symptoms, and were significantly more likely to maintain their recovery than women in usual care.

Preventing Depression

Interpersonal psychotherapy can also prevent postpartum depression in high-risk women (Zlotnick et al., 2006). Ninety-nine low-income pregnant women were randomly assigned to standard antenatal care or standard care plus interpersonal psychotherapy (Zlotnick et al., 2006). IPT's goal was to improve women's close, personal relationships; change their expectations about these relationships; build their social networks; and help them master their transition to motherhood. The intervention was four 60-minute group sessions during pregnancy, with one "booster" session after delivery. At 3 months postpartum, 4% of the intervention group became depressed compared to 20% of the control group.

The second study had a similar design. In this study, 205 women were randomized to IPT or treatment-as-usual conditions (Zlotnick et al., 2016). The women were all on public assistance, with a mean age of 23. Thirty-eight percent were Hispanic, and 23% Black. All were at high risk for postpartum depression. The intervention was four 90-minute group sessions during pregnancy, and one 50-minute individual "booster" at 2 weeks postpartum. At 6 months postpartum, 16% of the women in the intervention group were depressed compared to 31% of the control group. The researchers concluded that paraprofessionals could deliver a group intervention to at-risk women and reduce the risk of postpartum depression.

Clinical Takeaways

- Interpersonal psychotherapy is an effective treatment for both preventing and treating postpartum depression.
- At some point, interpersonal psychotherapy may supplant cognitive therapy as the frontline psychotherapy for postpartum depression.
- IPT can help partners understand depression and be more supportive.

18 Trauma-Informed Care and Trauma Treatment

Traumatic experiences are remarkably common among perinatal women. According to the US National Center for PTSD (2015), findings from a large national mental health study show that more than half of women will experience at least one traumatic event in their lives. The most common trauma for women is sexual assault or child sexual abuse, which affects one in three women. Women are also more likely to be neglected or abused in childhood, to experience domestic violence, or to witness violence. They may also have a traumatic birth. One in every nine of these women will develop PTSD.

KEY FINDINGS

- Trauma-informed care is designed to promote recovery and resilience for trauma survivors. All types of care should be safe and empowering.
- Psychotherapy is the frontline treatment for trauma. Medications can be used but are considered the second choice.
- Cognitive-processing therapy, prolonged exposure, eye-movement desensitization and reprocessing (EMDR), and cognitive-behavioral therapy are the forms of therapy most commonly used.
- Debriefing can be useful for mothers who have experienced birth trauma. It was most effective when mothers requested it several weeks after birth.

Trauma also increases the risk of depression during pregnancy and postpartum. In a study of 374 women recruited from a low-income, inner-city obstetrics clinic, 39% reported experiencing at least one traumatic event (Robertson-Blackmore et al., 2013). The most common events were child sexual abuse, having a close friend or family member experience violence, and the unexpected death or illness of someone close. Trauma-exposed women were up to four times more likely to be depressed during pregnancy. Depression during pregnancy can lead to many complications, including preterm birth (Kendall-Tackett, 2017).

Trauma survivors can be retraumatized in medical settings, which is why healthcare providers must be mindful of their needs. Even if you are not treating trauma, you can care for new mothers in a trauma-informed way, which recognizes their vulnerability. The US Substance Abuse Mental Health Services Administration (SAMHSA) (2015) outlined the principles of trauma-informed care.

In this case study, Anne reported her extensive history of child sexual assault. As an adult, she experienced numerous physical and mental health problems, including severe postpartum depression after the birth of her first child at 17. Yet the healthcare

DOI: 10.4324/9781003405092-22

system did not help her despite numerous opportunities to do so (Sigurdardottir & Halldorsdottir, 2018).

> Anne has constantly searched for ways to live with the physical consequences of CSA [child sexual abuse]. From a young age, she looked to the healthcare system for solutions without receiving adequate help, support, or understanding. . . . Anne has consistently asked her healthcare providers to recognize and validate her lived experience as a CSA survivor, as well as the connection these experiences have had on her chronic health conditions. However, the silence she experienced points to a systemic organizational problem in the education of healthcare professionals and healthcare professional socialization—treating only symptoms and not the underlying problem. . . . She told her doctors about the CSA, but they were silent, her lived experience of sexual violence was not discussed any further. . . . Anne asserts that what is most important is to be able to talk to people about the CSA, and be listened to, believed, and supported as a CSA survivor.
>
> (p. 12–13)

Anne's story highlights the need for care providers to be aware of trauma that their clients may have experienced and know resources that are available in their communities if their clients require follow-up care.

Trauma-Informed Care

Trauma-informed care (TIC) is a movement gaining momentum in healthcare but has not been widely adopted in maternity care. According to the US Substance Abuse and Mental Health Services Administration (SAMHSA, 2015), healthcare providers can promote the linkage to recovery and resilience for people impacted by trauma. Services and supports that are trauma-informed build on the best evidence available, consumer and family engagement, empowerment, and collaboration.

Trauma-informed care could be particularly relevant to community interventions, or any intervention administered by someone other than a mental health provider. The goal is to make healthcare safe for trauma survivors, but also to identify trauma and make appropriate referrals. According to SAMSHA (2015), a trauma-informed approach to care:

1. *Realizes* the widespread impact of trauma and understands potential paths for recovery.

For perinatal women, trauma increases the risk of depression, anxiety disorders, substance abuse, and PTSD. Trauma may also influence birth outcomes, including preterm delivery and birth-related PTSD.

2. *Recognizes* the signs and symptoms of trauma in clients, families, staff, and others involved with the system.

The perinatal period is a unique opportunity to recognize trauma and its effects. Trauma can be effectively treated, and helping mothers identify it can be the first step in their healing.

3. *Responds* by fully integrating knowledge about trauma into policies, procedures, and practices.

The effects of trauma are pervasive in the populations we serve. Yet healthcare providers often do not recognize its existence or the impact it can have on every area of a patient's life. We can counter this by recognizing trauma and instituting policies and practices that follow the principles of trauma-informed care.

4. Seeks to actively resist *re-traumatization*.

Birthing women are at high risk for experiencing medically induced trauma; the World Health Organization (2014) issued a statement calling for respectful care for women during labor and birth. During the postpartum period, high levels of oxytocin increase mothers' bonding with their babies but make them very attuned to social cues. Negative interactions with providers can have long-term effects (Uvnas-Moberg, 2015).

SAMHSA's Six Key Principles of Trauma-Informed Care

Key components of trauma-informed care are both organizational and clinical (Menschner & Maul, 2016). The organizational components include communicating about the transformation process, engaging patients in organizational planning, training clinical and non-clinical staff, preventing secondary trauma in staff, and hiring a trauma-informed workforce. The clinical components include involving patients in the treatment process, screening for trauma, training staff in trauma-informed practices, and referring clients to appropriate care with partnering organizations.

Menschner and Maul (2016) recommended asking patients to suggest organizational changes and serve alongside staff on oversight and advisory committees. Trauma-informed care should also include non-clinical staff and encourage them to treat clients in a welcoming manner, ensuring their safety while they are there. Even steps like monitoring who is in the building, making sure that parking lots are well-lit, and keeping noise levels down all help. In addition, patients need to feel that they can easily exit if they need to. The six key principles are not a prescribed set of practices or procedures. Rather, these principles are generalizable across multiple types of settings (Substance Abuse and Mental Health Services Administration (SAMHSA), 2015).

Safety

Safety is essential. When mothers do not feel safe, their fight-or-flight response is activated, which increases their symptoms. If mothers do not feel safe during labor, their contractions may stop. Fear postpartum can stop the flow of milk. The mechanism, in both cases, is the stress system blocking oxytocin, which will stop both labor contractions and milk ejection (Uvnas-Moberg, 2015). Fear can also compound their symptoms.

Trustworthiness and Transparency

Mothers need to feel they can trust their providers. TIC teaches providers how to gain mothers' trust and work with them most effectively.

Peer Support

Knowing people who have experienced similar things helps trauma survivors not feel so isolated. Peer support is important postpartum, and it is a key principle of TIC.

Collaboration and Mutuality

Mothers must feel that they are working with their healthcare providers as part of a team. They need to be involved in all aspects of their care. If they don't, they won't feel safe.

Empowerment, Voice, and Choice

All healthcare providers need to empower patients. When we "help" too much, mothers believe that they cannot do things on their own. True help allows mothers see the competencies they already possess.

Cultural, Historical, and Gender Issues

Every mother is unique. Listen. Ask questions. And assist where you can. Some suggest that "cultural humility" is a term preferable to "cultural competence." It implies an openness and willingness to learn what the families need, not what we think they need.

Treatments for Trauma

Psychotherapy and pharmacotherapy are effective treatments for PTSD. However, when both treatment options are available, the new US Veterans' Affairs/Department of Defense (VA/DoD) guidelines (2023) recommend psychotherapy over medications. Other organizations, such as the American Psychological Association (2017) and the British National Health Service (2022), recommend the same thing. The new US VA/DoD guidelines (2023) found strong evidence for individual, manualized, trauma-focused psychotherapies for PTSD: cognitive-processing therapy, eye-movement desensitization and reprocessing, and prolonged exposure. Other trauma treatments they list as "neither for nor against," citing current insufficient evidence. They also found insufficient evidence to recommend group or couples' therapy. These modalities are described next.

Cognitive-Processing Therapy (CPT)

Cognitive-processing therapy (CPT) is a specific type of cognitive-behavioral therapy that helps patients learn how to modify and challenge unhelpful beliefs related to the trauma. In so doing, the patient creates a new understanding and conceptualization of the traumatic event so that it reduces its ongoing negative effects on their life. CPT effectively reduces PTSD symptoms that developed after experiencing traumatic events, including child abuse, combat, rape, and natural disasters, and is generally delivered over 12 sessions.

The first part of treatment begins with psychoeducation about PTSD thoughts and emotions. Patients become more aware of automatic thoughts that may maintain PTSD symptoms. The patient writes an impact statement about why the event occurred and how it has influenced their beliefs about themselves, others, and the world.

The next step is more formal processing, where the patient writes a detailed account of their worst traumatic experience. They then read this statement in the next session to help them break the pattern of avoiding thoughts and feelings about the event. The therapist asks questions to try to identify unhelpful thoughts or maladaptive thinking. Once patients have developed the ability to identify and address unhelpful thinking, they can continue to modify their beliefs about traumatic events outside of treatment sessions to improve their functioning and quality of life. Therapists may focus on areas affected by trauma, such as safety, trust, power, control, and intimacy.

Prolonged Exposure

When people are traumatized, they develop a conditioned response that pairs the traumatic event with certain environmental cues (e.g., sights, sounds, smells) and bodily sensations: a process known as fear conditioning. In trauma-focused psychotherapy, there are two specific goals. The first is to unlearn the conditioned response that triggers PTSD symptoms. The second is to address PTSD-related cognitions about themselves and others.

Prolonged exposure (PE) is an intervention commonly used in cognitive-behavioral therapy to help individuals confront fears. PE is specifically designed to alleviate the conditioned emotional response of traumatic events to traumatic stimuli. After a traumatic event, patients naturally tend to avoid any memories of it, or any stimuli that reminds them of it. When patients avoid processing their trauma, it inhibits their recovery. Prolonged exposure teaches individuals to gradually approach trauma-related memories, feelings, and situations, helps patients master their fears, and counters the belief that they are weak or incompetent (National Center for PTSD, 2014). Most people want to avoid anything that reminds them of the trauma they experienced, but doing so reinforces their fear. By facing what they have been avoiding, a person can decrease symptoms of PTSD by learning that trauma-related memories and cues are not dangerous and do not need to be avoided.

Prolonged-exposure therapy begins when patients are asked to imagine the traumatic event. In a single session, patients repeatedly describe what happened, and their thoughts and feelings that occurred during the event (Foa & Cahill, 2002). During their narratives, patients are asked to report their level of distress every 10 minutes. If treatment is successful, patients can confront their traumatic pasts without triggering PTSD symptoms, especially intrusive thoughts or hyperarousal. This form of treatment is highly effective. However, van der Kolk (2002) cautions that too much exposure to traumatic memories can backfire and actually precipitate PTSD symptoms, such as hyperarousal and sensitization.

Exposure-based cognitive therapy is safe for treating anxiety disorders during pregnancy (Arch et al., 2012). Pregnant women have been excluded from previous studies because of the possible impact of the therapy on fetal programming. This risk has proven more hypothetical than actual, and the current state of knowledge is that the benefits (and risk associated with not treating or treating with medications) far outweigh possible risks of using exposure therapies during pregnancy. Arch et al. (2012) recommended that research on physiological markers during and after treatment with exposure therapies be conducted before recommending exposure treatments for all pregnant women with anxiety disorders. These include measures of cortisol, sympathetic functioning, and inflammatory response.

Eye-Movement Desensitization and Reprocessing (EMDR)

Eye-movement desensitization and reprocessing (EMDR) is a structured therapy that encourages the patient to briefly focus on the trauma memory while simultaneously experiencing bilateral stimulation (typically eye-movements), which reduces the vividness and emotion associated with the trauma memories. EMDR is based on the hypothesis that saccadic eye-movements can reprogram the brain and therefore can be used to help alleviate the emotional impact of trauma. (Saccadic eye-movements are the quick eye-movements that jump from one fixation point to another.)

During EMDR, clients imagine a traumatic memory, or any negative emotions associated with that memory. They are then asked to articulate a belief that is incompatible with their previous memory (e.g., on their personal worth). While clients remember this event, they are asked to use their eyes to follow the clinician's fingers that are making rapid movements. During treatment, clients are asked to rate the strength of both the traumatic memory and the counteracting positive beliefs (Friedman et al., 2009).

Studies have demonstrated that this method of treatment is effective; 50% to 70% of patients no longer met criteria for PTSD after receiving EMDR treatment. In contrast, only 20% to 50% of women who received supportive therapy no longer met PTSD criteria (Friedman, 2001). EMDR is an individual therapy typically delivered one to two times per week for a total of 6 to 12 sessions, although some people benefit from fewer sessions. Sessions can be conducted on consecutive days.

A case study of three women who suffered from posttraumatic-stress symptoms after their first births all underwent EMDR during a subsequent pregnancy (Stramrood et al., 2012). Following EMDR, all three patients had fewer PTS symptoms and felt more confident about their pregnancies and upcoming deliveries compared with before treatment. Even though all three women had complicated second deliveries, they remembered them positively. In addition, all three women were sufficiently confident following EMDR that they attempted a vaginal birth for their second delivery rather than requesting an elective cesarean.

Cognitive-Behavioral Therapy (CBT)

As I described in Chapter 16, cognitive-behavioral therapy focuses on the relationship among thoughts, feelings, and behaviors and notes how changes in any one domain can improve functioning in the other domains. Cognitive-behavioral therapy in trauma treatment is designed to counteract conditioned fear responses and to normalize abnormal thoughts, behaviors, and feelings of patients with PTSD.

CBT was effective in reducing trauma, anxiety, and depression symptoms in 105 mothers of preterm infants (Shaw et al., 2014). Mothers were randomly assigned to an either 6- or 9-session intervention based on CBT, or one session comprised of education about the NICU and parenting a preterm baby. The treatment was a manualized program of trauma-focused CBT, along with education about possible trauma triggers and parenting a preterm baby (including learning about vulnerable-child syndrome). It contained psychoeducation, cognitive restructuring, and trauma exposure. The mothers were assessed at 4 to 5 weeks and 6 months postpartum. They found that the 6-session intervention reduced trauma, anxiety, and depression symptoms compared to the control group. The mothers showed increased benefit of the intervention at 6 months. There was no difference between the 6- and 9-session interventions.

Medications

The current evidence base for PTSD psychopharmacology is strongest for the selective-serotonin reuptake inhibitors (SSRIs), sertraline and paroxetine, and the serotonin-norepinephrine reuptake inhibitor (SNRI) venlafaxine to treat PTSD (VA/DoD Clinical Practice Guideline, 2023). The new VA/DoD the guideline cite strong evidence for their use. But when given a choice between medications and psychotherapy, the guidelines recommend psychotherapy. However, they recognize that medications can reduce symptoms.

VA/DoD Practice Guidelines (2023) are neither for nor against amitriptyline, bupropion, buspirone, citalopram, desvenlafaxine, duloxetine, escitalopram, eszopiclone, fluoxetine, impramine, mirtazapine, lamotrigine, nefazodone, olanzapine, phenelzine, pregabalin, rivastigmine, topiramate, or quetiapine. They are also neither for nor against psychedelics, such as psilocybin, ayahuasca, or lysergic acid diethylamide (LSD).

The practice guidelines are "weak against" medications such as ketamine. They are "strongly against" benzodiazepines and cannabis to treat PTSD. Regarding ketamine, the guidelines acknowledged that it was known to be effective for other conditions (VA/DoD Clinical Practice Guideline, 2023) so could still be potentially considered for severe depression.

The British National Health Service (2022) recommended that medications only be used if:

- Someone did not have access to trauma-focused psychological treatment.
- Psychological treatment was not effective because there is ongoing trauma (e.g., domestic violence).
- The patient had not recovered with psychological treatment.
- The patient has a medical condition that affected their ability to benefit from psychological treatment (National Health Service, 2022).

Cannabis is of interest because people with PTSD may self-medicate with it to treat sleep problems, trauma symptoms, depression, anxiety, or chronic pain. However, the VA/DoD guidelines (2023) strongly recommend against it, citing possible negative psychiatric outcomes, such as depression, anxiety, psychosis, and substance misuse. They also cited issues about dose, route of administration, and legality, and issues such as CBD-to-THC ratio. Issues with perinatal women also include exposing the fetus to THC in utero and the infant via breastmilk (Volkow, 2019).

Complementary and Integrative Treatments for Trauma

Complementary and integrative treatments for PTSD are relatively new. These treatments have been incorporated into trauma treatment mainly because of patient demand (Kim, Schneider, et al., 2013). Even organizations that are relatively conservative with regard to treatment, such as the US Veterans Affairs, has recognized the demand for these modalities and are beginning to incorporate them into treatment for PTSD, albeit somewhat grudgingly (Williams et al., 2011). However, based on current evidence, the VA/DoD guidelines (2023) are neither for nor against these modalities. The following is a summary of findings on these techniques as trauma treatments.

Acupuncture

Recent studies have found acupuncture is effective in lessening PTSD symptoms. For example, in a randomized trial of 138 Chinese participants following the Wenchuan earthquake, researchers compared the effectiveness of electroacupuncture to paroxetine, treating participants for 12 weeks (Wang et al., 2012). After treatment, participants in the acupuncture group had lower levels of PTSD, depression, and anxiety than those in the paroxetine group at every assessment point (6 and 12 weeks, 3 and 6 months).

Mindfulness

Mindfulness can help trauma survivors develop more compassion toward themselves and others and become less critical of themselves. It reduced symptoms and changed behavior. It changed cognitions and improved self-management, relaxation, and acceptance (VA/DoD Clinical Practice Guideline, 2023). Mindfulness also reduced rumination over traumatic events, which increases PTSD symptoms (Kearney et al., 2013). Mindfulness could be used by itself or together with standard treatments (National Center for PTSD, 2010). The VA/DoD guidelines cited "weak evidence" for mindfulness to reduce stress but made no judgment for or against mindfulness added to other types of psychotherapy (such as mindfulness-based cognitive therapy).

Expressive Writing

Expressive writing is based on the work of James Pennebaker, who found that writing about stressful and traumatic life events for a brief period, even as little as 20 minutes per day over several days, resulted in significant reductions in depression, anxiety, PTSD symptoms, and health problems (Pennebaker, 2004). Expressive writing helps trauma survivors understand their experiences in a broader perspective and possibly derive meaning from them (Koopman et al., 2005).

Expressive writing has been helpful for those who have experienced combat or interpersonal violence. For example, one study included 47 women who had experienced severe intimate partner violence 5 years prior to the study. The women were randomly assigned to either expressive or neutral writing conditions (Koopman et al., 2005). The expressive writing group was asked to write about their most stressful or traumatic life experience. The neutral writing group was instructed to write about their daily schedules. There were four writing sessions that were 20 minutes each. The effects of expressive writing were strongest for women who were depressed, and it reduced the symptoms of depression in these women. A review also noted that expressive writing was effective for treating postpartum PTSD (Peeler et al., 2012).

A recent randomized trial examined the acceptability and feasibility of expressive writing for postpartum women (Crawley et al., 2018). The women were not screened for trauma as an inclusion criterion, so it is likely that women without trauma were included. Given that many of the women did not have trauma symptoms, the acceptance rate was low: 11% of the 854 women randomized to the intervention (expressive writing) or two control conditions (usual care or a control writing task). In addition, of the ones who accepted, the dropout rate was high: up to 68% at 6 months.

The intervention group was instructed to write expressively about a stressful event related to their pregnancy, birth, baby, or other life event and was asked to share their "deepest thoughts and feelings" for 15 minutes per day for 3 days. Only 29% of women in the expressive writing group complied. Mothers may have found this intervention intrusive or did not think it was safe to share these thoughts online or via mail. They were approached via a flyer and letter in their discharge packets. The most common topics were baby-related: baby's health, breastfeeding, crying baby, sleep, and baby's gender. The control writing condition was the same length of time, but mothers were asked to describe the room they were sitting in. Mothers in that group reported that the writing task was boring, and only 23% complied. They also reported that finding time to write was a barrier. However, women who did adhere to the intervention had stronger reactions (positive and negative) than mothers in the other writing group. In the qualitative portion, women indicated that they enjoyed writing even when they found it upsetting. The authors concluded that the feasibility of expressive writing as a universal self-help was low for women at 6 to 12 weeks postpartum but that it was an acceptable intervention to women who completed it.

Overall, I found the design of this study puzzling. It was offered to all postpartum women, but expressive writing is meant to be a specific intervention *for trauma*. For mothers who did not experience birth trauma, or other traumatic events, it would not seem relevant, so the low recruitment and compliance was not surprising. The mothers who did comply found it acceptable, which is good. But I would not recommend expressive writing as a universal treatment as it is more trauma specific.

Interventions Following Traumatic Childbirth

For women who have had traumatic births, timely intervention can lessen the severity of symptoms. Even short-term and low-key interventions can help. In one study, parents were interviewed regarding their distress following childbirth (Alder et al., 2006). If they were distressed, they were randomized into intervention and normal-care groups. The intervention was a 40- to 60-minute counseling session at 3 days, and a follow-up telephone call at 4 to 6 weeks postpartum. At 3 months, women in the intervention group had lower PTSD total symptoms than did women in the standard-care group. The intervention group also had lower depression and self-blame and higher confidence scores about having another baby. The authors recommended that interventions include counseling about subsequent pregnancies and birth options and strategies that help lower patient anxiety. A final component was relaxation training, including muscle relaxation and guided imagery.

Debriefing

Debriefing is an intervention designed to address traumatic birth. A midwife or another healthcare provider talks to women about their births. Women can ask questions and discuss any of their feelings of sadness, guilt, anger, or confusion. It was designed to help women process their experiences. In practice, findings have been mixed.

An Australian study included 917 women who had either been debriefed or had usual care following cesarean sections or assisted vaginal births (Small et al., 2000). The overall rates of depression were low in both groups (17% vs. 14% for debriefed vs. standard care, respectively). There were no significant differences between the groups, but a slightly *higher* percentage of debriefed women were depressed and in poorer health at 6 months postpartum compared with women with standard care. Mothers in the intervention group said that debriefing helped them, but the authors were concerned, concluded that debriefing was ineffective, and expressed caution.

In discussing the Small et al. study, Boyce and Condon (2001) noted that debriefing is used to prevent posttraumatic stress disorder, not depression. Given that, it is not surprising that this intervention did not lower depressive symptoms. In addition, women who had elective vs. emergency cesareans were grouped together, which may have obscured the findings. Finally, they questioned whether having a midwife do the debriefing if she had not been present at the birth was useful. How could they answer women's questions when they had not been there? They also pointed out that even though debriefing did not appear to be effective, women needed an opportunity to discuss their experiences.

A review on midwife-led debriefing found there was insufficient evidence on its effectiveness (Gamble et al., 2002). Methodological issues included the lack of a standardized debriefing intervention or comprehensive outcome variables. In addition, women's partners were often excluded. The authors concluded that a single-session intervention was insufficient to deal with the problem. Meades and colleagues (2011) raised similar concerns about the inconsistency in the use of the term *debriefing*, its purpose, the timing of the intervention, and what it entailed. Gamble and colleagues (2002) acknowledged that women may benefit from talking about their births. On the other hand, immediately after birth, the most deeply traumatized women may have been so numb that any intervention would not help.

Meades and colleagues (2011) worried that in getting rid of debriefing, we may have "thrown out the baby with the bathwater." They conducted a trial with 80 women who had given birth at the same hospital and met criterion A for PTSD: 46 women requested debriefing, and 34 women had not requested debriefing. PTSD symptoms lessened for women in both groups over time, but there were greater decreases in the women who requested debriefing. Debriefing did not lower depressive symptoms.

However promising these findings, some caution is in order. This study design did not account for pre-existing differences between the groups. For example, the debriefed group might have been higher in self-efficacy, reflected in the women's willingness to reach out for help. Self-efficacy increases the likelihood of recovering from trauma. Interestingly, they found that women in the debriefing group had worse appraisals of their births and lower social support than the non-debriefed group so were more at risk. Women waited, on average, 16.5 weeks before requesting debriefing—suggesting that previous studies may have debriefed too soon after birth for mothers to find it helpful. This study at least raises the possibility, however, that debriefing might be helpful *for some women*, suggesting that it might not be time to completely "throw out" the practice.

The Magical First Hour

Another recent study from Iran involved 84 new mothers diagnosed with traumatic childbirth (Abdollahpour et al., 2016). They were randomized into intervention (magical first hour) and control conditions. The magical first hour included allowing the baby to go through the 9 instinctive stages after birth rather than removing the infant from the mother: (1) the cry immediately after birth; (2) the baby relaxes, stops, and opens their eyes; (3) baby moves slightly upward and moves their head; (4) baby tries to locate the breast; (5) rest periods between other stages; (6) baby crawls to the breast; (7) baby licks the nipple, touches and massages the breast; (8) baby suckles at the breast; and (9) baby takes their first long sleep. The researchers "fully implemented" the 9 steps but were not more specific about what they did besides not removing the infant. Mothers in the control group had skin-to-skin contact with their babies as part of usual care.

PTSD was measured at three points postpartum: 2 weeks, 4 to 6 weeks, and 3 months (Abdollahpour et al., 2016). There were lower PTSD scores in the intervention groups across all three time points, although PTSD went down for mothers in both groups. It is not certain why the 9 steps would have this effect above and beyond normal skin-to-skin contact and breastfeeding, but the findings are of interest. They suggest that allowing mothers and infants time together after birth can lessen symptoms of PTSD, but why the 9 stages had a stronger effect than normal skin-to-skin contact and breastfeeding is unknown (e.g., did the infant stay with the mother for a longer period?). More findings are needed.

Clinical Takeaways

- All programs that work with new mothers should recognize that many will have been impacted by trauma.
- Even if your program does not provide counseling and trauma treatment, your program can be trauma-informed.
- Debriefing can help mothers who had traumatic births, but not immediately after. Debriefing is more effective if mothers request it when they are ready. Letting mothers know that debriefing is available when they need it is a way to support them.

Section V

Medications

19 Overview of Antidepressants

If mothers have moderate or severe depression, some practitioners believe medications are the only effective treatment because they change brain chemistry. When I wrote the first edition of this book, that view dominated the field. So much has changed. As I described in previous chapters, we now know that many non-pharmacological treatments also change brain chemistry. However, for some mothers, medications are still an essential part of treatment.

KEY FINDINGS

- Clinicians should listen to mothers' concerns about antidepressants. Mothers are more likely to cooperate, and take their medications, when they feel that their concerns have been heard.
- Typical antidepressants (tricyclics, selective-serotonin reuptake inhibitors, serotonin-norepinephrine reuptake inhibitors, and norepinephrine–dopamine inhibitors) are the most commonly prescribed. MAOIs come with significant restrictions on diet and can be dangerous when mixed with the wrong foods or over-the-counter medications.
- Antidepressants are most effective for vegetative symptoms.

Psychosocial Considerations about Antidepressants

For a treatment to work, mothers must be willing to participate. This is particularly true with antidepressants; they cannot work if mothers will not take them. In a review of 40 studies, Dennis and Chung-Lee (2006) found that women were often reluctant to take antidepressants, even after education about their relative safety. They worried about possible addiction, negative side effects, or harming their infants. There are also cultural considerations. Many communities distrust "White" medicine for a variety of reasons so reject antidepressants as an option. Practitioners need to have open conversations with patients about their fears and concerns while also recognizing that some will still refuse. In which case, other options should be considered.

On the issue of whether medications are necessary, I appreciate Dr. David Burns's perspective. He is a psychiatrist so could prescribe medication for all his patients. He is also the author of one of the best self-help books in the field on cognitive therapy: *Feeling good: The new mood therapy* (Burns, 1999). He acknowledges that medications are useful, and noted about 40% of his patients benefited from a short course of antidepressants to help them "get over the hump." However, he does not believe that all patients need to be on them or that most people need to be on them for the rest of their lives.

DOI: 10.4324/9781003405092-24

Angelotta and Wisner (2017) noted that the decision to use antidepressants depends on the mother's response to them, the probability of adverse fetal effects, and the mother's characteristics and values. The goal is complete remission of symptoms so that we do not expose the infant to both depression and medication. Mothers need an optimal dose, which treats symptoms yet has tolerable side effects. Interestingly, they noted that pregnant women require higher doses than they do postpartum because of cytochrome P450 (CYP450), an enzyme that reduces the concentration of serotonin in the plasma, because it is metabolized more quickly. As a result, pregnant women are often undermedicated.

Selecting Which Medication to Use

When considering whether a medication is necessary, think about which symptoms you want to address. Also consider the mother's history with antidepressants.

Symptoms That Antidepressants Address

Antidepressants are most helpful for vegetative symptoms. These include sleep disturbance, including early-morning awakening, decreased sleep efficiency, frequent awakenings through the night, and possibly hypersomnia; appetite disturbance, eating too much or too little; fatigue; decreased sex drive (a normal symptom postpartum); diurnal variations in mood (e.g., feeling worse in the morning); restlessness or agitation; impaired concentration; and "pronounced anhedonia," or the inability to experience pleasure (Preston et al., 2022).

Mother's History

Did the mother have previous success with antidepressants? Her history predicts whether she will respond to medication. Were the side effects intolerable? Common side effects include sedation, weight gain, orthostatic hypotension, and sexual dysfunction. What other medications is the patient currently taking? Possible drug–drug interactions should be considered. What does the medication cost? Newer medications are considerably more expensive than the older antidepressants that are available in generic form. Mothers who are potentially suicidal need to avoid certain types of antidepressants (tricyclics or MAOIs) that can be lethal in overdose or in combination with certain foods.

Depression Severity and Risk/Benefit Analysis in Treatment Decisions

Antidepressants raise safety concerns with perinatal women because infants are also exposed. Depression severity figures into the balance of risk associated with their use. When a mother's depression is severe, the benefits most likely outweigh the risks. The risk/benefit analysis is less clear among patients with milder depression. Does the benefit outweigh the risk in these patients? Freeman (2007) suggested that non-pharmacologic choices may be most appropriate for women with mild depression. However, if depression is moderate to severe, or if a mother has a history of depression, medications may still be the best first choice. I describe risk/benefit analyses in more detail in the next chapter.

Typical Antidepressants

Preston et al. (2022) group antidepressants into three main categories: typical, atypical, and monoamine oxidase inhibitors (MAOIs). All increase the availability of neurotransmitters, such as serotonin-norepinephrine and dopamine. The selective-serotonin reuptake inhibitors (SSRIs) are the medications most prescribed for pregnant and postpartum women. They are part of the typical antidepressant class, which also includes the older tricyclics. I describe the atypical antidepressants in Chapter 22.

Tricyclics

Tricyclic antidepressants (TCAs) are an older class of antidepressants with a solid track record. TCAs include nortriptyline and amitriptyline (Osborne et al., 2014). They work but have side effects that people do not like, so patient compliance can be a problem (Kroska & Stowe, 2020). TCAs have another serious drawback: they can be lethal in too large a dose. If these medications are used, patients must be closely monitored. If a patient has any risk of suicide, safer choices are fluoxetine, sertraline, paroxetine, or bupropion (Preston et al., 2022).

Selective-Serotonin Reuptake Inhibitors (SSRIs)

SSRIs are the most prescribed antidepressants for new mothers and include fluoxetine (Prozac), sertraline (Zoloft), paroxetine (Paxil), citalopram (Celexa), and escitalopram (Lexapro). They are considered a first-line medication treatment and have low risk of possible overdose and less severe side effects than tricyclics (Kroska & Stowe, 2020). As their name implies, they work specifically on serotonin receptors, and their dosing schedule is less complex. SSRIs are effective for approximately 70% of patients (Preston et al., 2022).

Two SSRIs, sertraline and paroxetine, are also FDA-approved for the treatment of PTSD, particularly re-experiencing, avoidance, numbing, and hyperarousal symptoms (Kelmendi et al., 2017). A major issue with SSRIs are their sexual side effects (di Scalea et al., 2009; Preston et al., 2022). However, some sexual symptoms may be due to depression and not the medication. A study of 70 postpartum women with major depression compared two antidepressants, nortriptyline (a tricyclic) or sertraline (an SSRI), in an 8-week clinical trial (di Scalea et al., 2009). At the beginning of the trial, 73% complained of three or more sexual concerns. By 8 weeks, only 37% mentioned sexual concerns. Those whose depression remitted reported significantly fewer sexual concerns than did women whose depression did not remit. This finding was independent of the medication type. The authors concluded that sexual concerns may be more a function of depression rather than a side effect of a particular medication. This suggests that mothers who continue to report sexual side effects may still be depressed and should be reassessed.

Another issue with SSRIs are their potential interactions with other medications. When using SSRIs, take a careful history of other prescription, over-the-counter, and herbal medications the patient is taking. SSRIs can be dangerous if taken with MAO inhibitors, non-sedating antihistamines, tricyclic antidepressants, and lithium because they may increase levels of each. There can also be problems if they are taken with carbamazepine and St. John's wort (Preston et al., 2022). If mothers want to switch from an SSRI to St. John's wort, the washout period is 5 days.

Serotonin-Norepinephrine Reuptake Inhibitors

Newer antidepressants are serotonin-norepinephrine reuptake inhibitors (SNRI), such as venlafaxine and mirtazapine. Mirtazapine is most useful as an add-on medication to enhance the effectiveness of other antidepressants, such as bupropion and venlafaxine, in cases of severe or treatment-resistant depression. Desvenlafaxine is the synthetic form of the major active metabolite of venlafaxine. A study of the milk and plasma of 10 depressed breastfeeding mothers revealed relative infant dose of 4.8% for all 10 mothers, and 5.3% for the exclusively breastfeeding mothers (Rampono et al., 2011). The author noted that safety data are encouraging, but urge further studies before recommending it as a monotherapy for mothers.

Norepinephrine–Dopamine Inhibitors

Bupropion is a norepinephrine–dopamine reuptake inhibitor that is also used for smoking cessation (under the brand name Zyban) (Preston et al., 2022). Unlike the other antidepressants, it works on dopamine receptors and is often used as an add-on medication when SSRIs lead to an incomplete response. Bupropion is helpful when the primary symptoms are hypersomnia, fatigue, and low energy. It does not cause sexual dysfunction, weight gain, or sleepiness and is sometimes prescribed to counter these effects in SSRIs.

Monoamine Oxidase Inhibitors (MAOIs)

MAOIs are very effective antidepressants. They may be prescribed for refractory or atypical depressions but are not widely used because of their strict dietary restrictions and potentially lethal side effects. When taking these medications, patients cannot eat or drink anything with tyramine, a by-product of bacterial fermentation. Tyramine is common in foods, such as red wine and cheese. MAOIs with tyramine can cause a hypertensive crisis or death. Patients also need to avoid many over-the-counter products, such as cold medications and pain relievers. MAOIs include phenelzine, isocarboxazid, and tranylcypromine.

These medications are enjoying a surprising renaissance of use because if the dietary restrictions are observed, some practitioners feel they are safer than tricyclics and have fewer side effects (Kiecolt-Glaser et al., 2010). (Amazing, in my mind, considering that possible *death* is one of the side effects.) **These medications are the only antidepressants that are contraindicated for breastfeeding mothers** (Hale, 2021). MAOIs may cause permanent changes in the baby, and the risk never outweighs the benefits.

Phases of Depression Management with Medications

Managing depression with medication has three main phases: acute, continuation, and maintenance (Preston et al., 2022). Knowing about the phases of management can help you communicate a treatment plan, chart any discussion of medications with mothers, as well as discuss stopping medications or using non-drug treatments.

Acute Phase

The acute phase is the first 6 to 12 weeks of the depressive episode, which begins with the first dose and lasts until the patient is asymptomatic (Preston et al., 2022). The objectives are to rapidly reduce symptoms, monitor patients for suicide risk, and evaluate the medication's effectiveness. If the medication is not effective, there are two possible explanations: the dose is not high enough, or the treatment has not been long enough for an adequate response. Assessments should include an evaluation of symptoms, work or school productivity, and improvement in interpersonal relationships.

Talk to patients about what they should expect from the medications. Patients who are adequately educated are more likely to comply with treatments when they understand side effects and have realistic expectations about what medications will do. Preston et al. (2022) recommend giving patients the following information.

1. Medications may take 10 to 21 days before you notice a difference in symptoms.
2. When symptoms do improve, it is likely that they will be the ones with a biological basis, such as sleep disturbance. They may not help with psychologically based symptoms, such as self-esteem.
3. Treatment is working when you are sleeping better, have less daytime fatigue, and have some improvement in emotional control.
4. There may be side effects, but these can be managed.
5. The total length of time to be on antidepressants varies for everyone.
6. Antidepressants are not addictive.

Continuation Phase

The continuation phase lasts from 4 to 9 months. The objective is to prevent a relapse of symptoms, which can occur if treatment is terminated during this time (Lesperance & Frasure-Smith, 2000). If symptoms have not improved, or if the patient has relapsed, re-evaluate both the diagnosis and patient compliance. Are comorbid conditions keeping treatments from being effective? Is the medication effective, or should another be tried? Is the patient complying with treatment and taking the medications as directed?

A larger dose may be needed in some cases, or the patient may need to be on the medication for a longer period. The most common mistake is to under-medicate depressed patients (Preston et al., 2022). This is also true for patients with anxiety, who often require substantially higher dosages for symptoms to remit. Generally, the length of an adequate trial is 4 to 6 weeks. If the medication is not effective after that time, another medication should be considered, or an additional medication could be added to the regimen.

Maintenance Phase

This phase should be initiated for patients who have had multiple episodes of depression or who have particularly severe or difficult-to-treat episodes and are therefore at high risk of recurrence. This phase may be for life in some patients, particularly those who have had three or more episodes of major depression.

The Anti-Inflammatory Effects of Antidepressants

In addition to influencing levels of neurotransmitters, antidepressants are also anti-inflammatory, which partially explains why they work (Leonard, 2010; Maes et al., 2009). Maes and colleagues (2009) noted that when researchers only focused on neurotransmitters, they missed something critical about the way antidepressants worked. Antidepressants influence serotonin-norepinephrine, but they also lower inflammation. If you understand inflammation's role, you know that antidepressants can only be partially effective if they do not adequately address it. To increase their effectiveness, you can add an anti-inflammatory, such as a COX-2 inhibitors (like Celebrex) or an omega-3 fatty acid (Kiecolt-Glaser et al., 2015; Maes et al., 2009; Pace et al., 2007).

But antidepressants also lower inflammation on their own. SSRIs decreased C-reactive protein in cardiac patients with major depression (O'Brien et al., 2006). Fluoxetine and desipramine lowered inflammation in two animal models of human disease: septic shock and asthma (Roumestan et al., 2007). The authors concluded that antidepressants are directly anti-inflammatory and can treat inflammatory conditions. An in vitro study of inflammation was designed to test whether venlafaxine would modulate the inflammatory response (Vollmar et al., 2008). In an astroglia-microglia co-culture, they demonstrated that venlafaxine was anti-inflammatory and decreased IL-6 and IL-8. This understanding led to several important discoveries, such as using antidepressants to treat autoimmune and inflammatory conditions so that patients can use lower dosages of steroids.

Clinical Takeaways

- Antidepressants are an important part of the treatment arsenal for women with post-partum depression and related conditions.
- All but one type (MAOIs) are compatible with breastfeeding. They can be combined with other modalities (except for St. John's wort) to give mothers additional tools to reduce inflammation, improve their sleep, cope with future life stresses, and increase their sense of competence and self-efficacy.
- Managing depression with medications includes three phases: acute, continuation, and maintenance. All phases involve re-assessing depression to see if the medication is working. Many clinicians do not follow up, but it is a key part of care.

20 Antidepressants for Pregnant or Breastfeeding Women

Is it safe for pregnant or breastfeeding women to use antidepressants? Mothers and clinicians are both understandably concerned. Yonkers (2007) describes this dilemma and notes that clinicians have to make decisions, sometimes with insufficient data. This leaves clinicians in a "gray zone" of whether to treat or not (Chaudron, 2007).

> The absence of sufficient data is not the result of a lack of interest among researchers but derives largely from the ethical or practical issues that make research in this area difficult.
>
> (p. 1,459)

No decision is risk-free when treating pregnant and breastfeeding women but involves balancing different types of risk (Malm et al., 2015; Newport et al., 2002). Caution is appropriate. During pregnancy, is the risk of exposing the fetus to medication higher than the risk of mothers' untreated depression, which increases the risk of preterm birth? For postpartum women, is the risk of exposing an infant to medication via breastmilk higher than the risks associated with formula? These are examples of risks that need to be considered.

KEY FINDINGS

- Antidepressants during pregnancy increase the risk for birth defects but affect less than 1% of infants.
- Continuous antidepressant use during pregnancy can increase the risk of preterm birth to a level comparable to untreated depression.
- Third-trimester SSRI or tricyclic exposure can cause discontinuation syndrome. Discontinuation syndrome is more likely if mothers took medications with shorter half-lives.
- The risk of not breastfeeding usually exceeds the risk of exposing infants to the medication via breastfeeding.
- Medications with high molecular weight and protein binding are less likely to transfer into breastmilk.

Physicians may avoid prescribing antidepressants during pregnancy. A study of 61 Australian general practitioners (GPs) and Canadian family practice physicians found that healthcare providers from both countries were confused about the safety of antidepressants during pregnancy because of the many conflicting reports (Bilszta et al., 2011).

DOI: 10.4324/9781003405092-25

Forty-two percent of general practitioners believed that they were safe vs. 83% of family practitioners. Further, family practitioners were more likely than the GPs to believe that antidepressants were safe for the fetus (10% vs. 48%), and they had more confidence about using them during pregnancy (33% vs. 57%).

A study analyzing Tennessee Medicaid data, which included 228,876 singleton pregnancies, found that prescriptions for depressed pregnant women decreased following US and Canadian public health advisory warnings about the risk of antidepressant-related perinatal complications (Bobo et al., 2014). Prescription rates dropped more quickly for SSRIs than other types. Before the warnings were issued, prescription rate increased steadily. After the advisories, prescription rates dropped, but antidepressants were still prescribed.

In Utero Effects of Antidepressants

Prenatal exposure to antidepressants increases the risk of fetal complications, which are statistically rare but still need to be thoroughly discussed with the mother. Among the complications are possible preterm birth, congenital heart problems, and behavioral outcomes in infants and children.

Antidepressants and Preterm Birth

Untreated depression increases the risk of preterm birth, but so do antidepressants. In a study of depressed pregnant women, more than 20% of infants with continuous exposure to selective-serotonin reuptake inhibitors (SSRIs) during pregnancy were delivered preterm (Wisner et al., 2009). This study included 238 women who were assessed at 20, 30, and 36 weeks' gestation. The patients were divided into three groups: no depression, no SSRI exposure (n=131); SSRI exposure that was either continuous (n=48) or partial (n=23); or untreated major depression that was either continuous (n=14) or partial (n=22). Thirty-four percent took sertraline, 25% fluoxetine, 23% citalopram or escitalopram, and 18% other medications. By the end of the study, 20% of the infants with continuous SSRI exposure were preterm. However, 20% of mothers with continuous *untreated depression* had preterm births. The rate of preterm birth among the non- or partially exposed groups ranged from 4% to 9%.

A population study of all singleton births in Finland between 1996 and 2000 compared pregnancies exposed to SSRIs (N = 15,729), women with psychiatric illness who did not take SSRIs (N = 9,652), and women with no SSRI exposure and no psychiatric illness (N = 31,394) (Malm et al., 2015). Mothers on SSRIs had lower risk of late preterm birth, very preterm birth, and cesarean section compared to mothers with psychiatric illness with no SSRI exposure. Offspring of mothers with non-medicated psychiatric illness and mothers who took SSRIs were both at increased risk of adverse pregnancy outcomes.

In British Columbia, Canada, a large population study (N = 119,547) compared SSRI-exposed infants to infants of depressed, untreated mothers and infants of non-depressed mothers. The percentage of SSRI-exposed infants ranged from 2% to 5% over the 39-month recruitment period. Birthweight and gestational age were significantly less for the SSRI-exposed infants compared with infants of untreated depressed mothers. The medications used were paroxetine (44.7%), fluoxetine (27.2%), sertraline (25.6%), fluvoxamine (4.6%) and citalopram (3.3%) (Oberlander et al., 2006).

A study from the Netherlands of 7,696 pregnant women found that infants of mothers with untreated depression had reduced body and head growth in utero (El Marroun et al., 2012). The mothers taking SSRIs during pregnancy had fewer depressive symptoms, but their offspring were twice as likely to be preterm. Small infant head size predicts behavioral and internalizing problems, such as anxiety and ADHD. However, they noted that *for some women*, the benefits of SSRIs outweighed their risk.

Timing of medication exposure influences the complications associated with their use. First- and third-trimester exposures are the times of greatest concern.

First-Trimester Exposure

A prospective study collected data from women whose babies were born between 1995 and 2003. There were 200 neonates exposed to antidepressants in utero, and 1,200 controls (Maschi et al., 2008). There were three groups that differed in the timing of when they took antidepressants: before conception and during first trimester, during the second and third trimesters, and before conception and during the entire pregnancy. The most frequently used medications were paroxetine (58 cases), fluoxetine (32 cases), and amitriptyline (26 cases). Consistent with previous studies, exposed infants had increased risk for preterm birth. This was particularly true for those chronically exposed.

Of 200 exposed infants, 14 experienced adverse events, and 3 required NICU/SCN admission (Maschi et al., 2008). No significant difference was found after adjusting for prematurity, birthweight, and sex of the infant, and no significant effects were found by medication type. Three cases (5%) of neonatal complications were reported with paroxetine exposure, one of which required admission to the NICU. In contrast, in the non-exposed group, 17 had complications (5%), six of which required NICU admission. One case of cardiac malformation was reported following paroxetine exposure in the first trimester, and a total of 2% of the control group had malformations, none of which were cardiac malformations. A major limitation of these findings is that data were collected via maternal interview and therefore may have underreported, especially the minor effects.

The results of the Sloane Epidemiology Center Birth Defects Study also confirmed that SSRIs do not significantly increase the risk of birth defects overall. They included three birth defects in their study: craniosynostosis, omphalocele, and heart defects (Louik et al., 2007). Sertraline increased the risk of omphalocele and septal defects, and paroxetine increased the risk of a heart defect: right ventricular outflow tract obstruction. Even with these odds ratios, only 2% to 5% of infants with these defects were exposed to SSRIs in the first trimester. The authors concluded that the overall risk of having a child affected by SSRI use was 0.2%.

First-trimester exposure may also increase the risk of miscarriage. In a sample of 937 pregnant women exposed to antidepressants before and during early pregnancy, there were 122 spontaneous abortions, including three ectopic pregnancies (Einarson et al., 2009). In their comparison group of 937 non-exposed pregnant women, there were 75 spontaneous abortions and no ectopic pregnancies. Logistic regression indicated that antidepressant exposure, and prior spontaneous abortion, were the risk factors for current miscarriage. The authors concluded that antidepressant exposure in the first trimester is associated with a small but statistically significant risk of miscarriage. The authors urged caution in interpreting these results because decisions to medicate must also consider the effects of untreated depression.

Third-Trimester Exposure and Discontinuation Syndrome

In neonates, third-trimester exposure is related to SSRI withdrawal or "discontinuation syndrome" (Hale et al., 2010). Discontinuation syndrome includes tremors, jitteriness, excessive crying, sleep disturbances, acrocyanosis, tachypnea, temperature instability, and irritability (Fuemmeler et al., 2012). When comparing exposed and non-exposed infants, the rates of complications were 14% for neonatal respiratory distress (vs. 8%), 9% for jaundice (vs. 8%), and 4% for feeding problems (vs. 2%). The length of hospital stay was significantly longer for exposed infants, suggesting that SSRI exposure created an independent effect. The authors concluded that exposure to prenatal SSRIs increased risk of low birthweight and respiratory distress, even when maternal illness severity was accounted for (Oberlander et al., 2006). These findings were contrary to what they predicted. They hypothesized that reducing depression would lessen adverse neonatal complications associated with maternal depression. They also noted that when mothers were inadequately medicated, infants were exposed to SSRIs and depressed maternal mood, which compounded the negative effect for these outcomes.

A convenience sample of 930 women who had taken antidepressants while breastfeeding responded to an advertisement on a breastfeeding-and-medication forum on a website (Hale et al., 2010). Five hundred twenty-seven of these women had also taken antidepressants while pregnant. The women completed an online survey reporting on symptoms their infants experienced in the immediate postpartum period. Most women reported that their infants never experienced discontinuation syndrome. Twenty-five percent reported that their infants were irritable, 17% reported inconsolable crying, 14% had low body temperature, and 15% had trouble eating and sleeping. Mothers who took antidepressants during pregnancy and while breastfeeding were 2 to 8 times more likely to report discontinuation symptoms than women who took them only while breastfeeding. In addition, if mothers took antidepressants with shorter half-lives (meaning, that the level dropped more quickly after delivery), their infants were more likely to have discontinuation syndrome

A study of 997 infants and 987 mothers sought to prospectively investigate the effects of antidepressants on neonates during the third trimester (Kallen, 2004). The medications used included tricyclic antidepressants, such as clomipramine and amitriptyline, and SSRIs, including citalopram, paroxetine, fluoxetine, and sertraline. Exposure increased risk for preterm birth and low birthweight. After exposure to antidepressants, especially tricyclics, there was an increased risk for low Apgar scores, respiratory distress, neonatal convulsions, and hypoglycemia. Infant outcomes after exposure to paroxetine were not worse than exposure to other SSRIs.

Childhood Effects of Pre- and Postnatal SSRI Exposure

Two studies examined longer-term effects of pre-and postnatal exposure to SSRIs. Both studies included the same cohort of patients and were designed to assess "behavioral teratogenicity" that may have occurred in the wake of SSRI exposure in utero and via breastmilk. Behavioral teratogenicity included internalizing and externalizing behaviors as indicated on the Child Behavior Checklist. Internalizing behaviors included emotional reactivity, depression, anxiety, irritability, and withdrawal (Misri et al., 2006). Externalizing behaviors included hyperactivity, impulsiveness, noncompliance, verbal and physical aggression, disruptive acts, emotional outbursts, and lack of task persistence, and problem-solving (Oberlander et al., 2007).

In these studies, 22 SSRI-exposed infants were compared to 14 non-exposed infants. Of the 22 depressed mothers, 5 were taking fluoxetine, 14 paroxetine, and 3 sertraline. Nine of these women were also taking olanzapine. The exposure to the medication was substantial, averaging 181 days of prenatal exposure, 60 days postnatal for SSRIs, and 41 days postnatal for olanzapine (Misri et al., 2006; Oberlander et al., 2007). Amazingly, mothers in this study remained symptomatic even after being treated for depression: 64% still had anxiety symptoms, and 73% had depressive symptoms. At the 4-year visit, 59% had anxiety symptoms, and 50% had depressive symptoms (Misri et al., 2006).

Regarding medication exposure, there were no significant differences in either parent or caregiver ratings of internalizing behaviors (Misri et al., 2006). Independent raters also rated the child's behavior in a laboratory setting, where they were blind to their medication status, and there were no differences between exposed and non-exposed groups. When the entire cohort was measured, mothers were more likely to report symptoms in their children when they were anxious or depressed. This was not true for teacher ratings, and the relationship remained, even after prenatal exposure was added to the model. Maternal mood was a better predictor of mother-reported internalizing behaviors than prenatal medication exposure.

Similarly, there was no difference at age 4 in externalizing behaviors between the exposed and non-exposed groups (Oberlander et al., 2007). Current maternal depression and anxiety predicted externalizing at age 4 more than prenatal medication exposure. Umbilical cord blood levels were associated with externalizing behaviors at 4 years, but once current maternal depression was added to the model, it only accounted for 11% of the variance in behavioral outcomes. Exposure was related to the child's lower persistence in the laboratory observation. Poor neonatal adaptation predicted increased aggression at age 4. Current maternal stress and depression more accurately predicted externalizing behaviors, regardless of prenatal depressed mood or medication exposure. This study was the first to consider the dual role of prenatal SSRI exposure and current maternal mood.

Another study of 166 mother–infant dyads compared mothers with major depression who took SSRIs during pregnancy (N = 68) and non-exposed controls (N = 98) (Santucci et al., 2014). Prenatal SSRI exposure had no impact on scores from the Psychomotor Development Index, the Mental Development Index, or the Behavioral Rating Scale. There was a significant difference in Psychomotor Development scores at 26 weeks for SSRI-exposed infants. However, this difference disappeared by 52 weeks. The authors concluded that the effects of SSRIs on psychomotor development may be transitory.

In contrast, a more recent study found that prolonged use of SSRIs during pregnancy was related to delayed fine and gross motor development, even after adjusting for mothers' symptoms of depression and anxiety (Handal et al., 2016). SSRI use was only weakly associated with delays in motor development. The authors concluded that these delays were not clinically important. Their findings were based on a prospective population-based pregnancy cohort study from Norway. Three hundred and eighty-one women reported using SSRIs while pregnant (only 0.7% of the total study population), and 159 had prolonged SSRI use.

In another analysis from the same data set, Skurtveit and colleagues (2014) found that prolonged use of SSRIs during pregnancy was associated with lower language competence for the infants at age 3. These findings were independent of maternal depression and anxiety during pregnancy. Postpartum depression did not influence the results. Although statistically significant, very few children had clinically impaired language development.

A birth cohort study from Denmark found no increase in behavioral problems in children exposed to SSRIs in utero (Grzeskowiak et al., 2015). Their sample included 210 pregnant women who took SSRIs, 231 depressed women who did not take antidepressants, and healthy controls who were neither depressed nor took SSRIs (N = 48,737). The researchers found no association between prenatal antidepressant use and problem behavior, hyperactivity, or peer problems at age 7. Antidepressant exposure was related to emotional symptoms and conduct problems. However, these associations attenuated when mother's antenatal mood was considered. Untreated prenatal depression increased risk for all the behavior problems that were included in this study. The authors concluded that prenatal antidepressant exposure was not associated with behavior problems in exposed children at age 7.

Breastfeeding and Medications

Regarding breastfeeding, any risk/benefit analysis must weigh the risk of infant exposure to mothers' medications via breastmilk vs. the risk of *not breastfeeding*, which can be considerable. The oft-made recommendation to use formula "just to be safe" does not consider the risk associated with non-breastmilk substitutes. In most cases, the risk associated with breastfeeding on medication is still less than using breastmilk substitutes.

When considering whether a medication is risky to use while breastfeeding, there are two key questions we need to ask: Does the medication pass into breastmilk? And does medication in milk affect infants? (Kendall-Tackett & Hale, 2010). The risk of exposure via breastmilk is significantly lower with breastfeeding than it is during pregnancy, and some medications are less likely than others to transfer into the milk.

Breastfeeding mothers will be more amenable to taking antidepressants if they understand how much transfers into milk and how they can minimize their infants' exposure. Unfortunately, practitioners sometimes communicate that breastfeeding is "no big deal" and that it can be easily discarded. That attitude fails to acknowledge what the mother wants to do, which often leads to them ignoring providers' advice. I know several mothers who were prescribed antidepressants, brought them home, and dumped them in the toilet. The practitioners who prescribed them assumed that they had treated the patient. In reality, they had not.

In a study from France, 405 new mothers were asked about the acceptability of treatments for depression, including psychotherapy by consultation, psychotherapy by home visit, and antidepressants (Chabrol et al., 2004). Psychotherapy was more acceptable than antidepressants, even after mothers learned that about the relatively small amount of medication in their breastmilk. However, what the researchers said to the mothers may explain the findings. What follows is a partial account of what they told mothers in their study.

> However, the effects of the antidepressants on the developing brain of the child and the long-term consequences are unknown. In the case of breastfeeding, it is therefore recommended not to prescribe antidepressants except in the cases where the advantages can clearly be shown to outweigh the potential risks.
>
> (p. 7)

No wonder mothers were reluctant! While we do not have all the answers, we can make some reasoned conclusions.

Does Medication Cross into Breastmilk?

Since psychotropic medications are lipid-soluble, they pass into breastmilk via passive diffusion, some more heavily than others. Relative infant dose (RID) is a widely accepted method to estimate infant exposure to mother's medication, which is calculated by dividing infant dose by the average maternal dose. Medications with high molecular weights or high protein binding are less likely to pass into milk. They are generally considered compatible with breastfeeding if the RID is less than 10% (Kronenfeld et al., 2017).

Of all antidepressants studied, sertraline has been studied the most. These studies consistently reveal that sertraline is virtually undetectable in infant plasma most of the time (Kroska & Stowe, 2020). Similarly, paroxetine transfers in minimal amounts. Paroxetine is not recommended during pregnancy but is one of the better choices for breastfeeding. In contrast, fluoxetine transfers to infants and, because of its long half-life, could accumulate in them. Because of these characteristics, it is less preferable, particularly with newborns (Fuemmeler et al., 2012; Kendall-Tackett & Hale, 2010).

A meta-analysis of 67 studies of antidepressant levels in breastfeeding infants pooled data from 337 research cases, including 238 infants (Markowitz & Weissman, 2004). The researchers analyzed data on 15 different antidepressants and their major metabolites and found that they all were detectable in the breastmilk with varying amounts. The authors indicated that there are many factors that influence transfer of medication to infants via breastmilk. Fluoxetine was more likely to accumulate in breastfeeding infants. There was also a case report of an infant with no prenatal exposure having symptoms following exposure to citalopram via breastfeeding. This infant's RID was 13% of the average maternal dose (Markowitz & Weissman, 2004).

Regarding long-term effects, low or undetectable infant plasma concentrations do not mean no long-term effects, but studies with asymptomatic infants are reassuring (Markowitz & Weissman, 2004). Prenatal exposure provides a "loading dose" that far exceeds any exposure from breastmilk and can distort findings regarding exposure via breastmilk. In addition, studies often fail to account for other confounds, such as maternal smoking or alcohol use, both of which can affect infant metabolism (Markowitz & Weissman, 2004).

The Bottom Line

Breastfeeding infants exposed to paroxetine and sertraline are unlikely to have detectable or elevated plasma drug levels. In contrast, infants exposed to fluoxetine had higher levels of exposure, especially if they had been exposed prenatally. These findings raise some concerns, but fluoxetine is not contraindicated. Fluoxetine is rapidly metabolized into long half-life active metabolites, and the amount in breastmilk is higher than in other SSRIs (Kronenfeld et al., 2017). Citalopram may lead to elevated levels in some infants, but more data are needed. Although these medications appear safe for the majority of infants, case studies have noted some adverse effects. Therefore, breastfeeding mothers should be advised to watch for any signs of adverse reactions, including irritability, poor feeding, or uneasy sleep.

Escitalopram produces low levels in milk and does not cause harm to breastfed infants. One study of 8 women examined the transfer of escitalopram and its metabolite into breastmilk (Kristensen et al., 2006). Mothers had been taking the medication for an average of 55 days. The total relative infant dose for escitalopram and its metabolite was 5.3% of the maternal weight-adjusted dose (3.9% for escitalopram; 1.7% for desmethylescitalopram). The levels were undetectable in four infants, and at very low levels in two others. Based on the infant dose calculations, the authors concluded that escitalopram is preferred to citalopram and is safe for breastfeeding women.

The American Academy of Pediatrics identified three tricyclic antidepressants (clomipramine, doxepin, and nortriptyline) as medications of concern for breastfeeding infants, particularly when used long-term. The concerns were mostly regarding active metabolites and longish half-lives of the medications and their metabolites (Kronenfeld et al., 2017).

The SNRIs have similar safety profiles to the SSRIs, but there are fewer studies available. Due to lack of safety data, they are considered second-line treatments for depression in breastfeeding mothers. Venlafaxine is the most studied of this class and might be the preferred. Desvenlafaxine offers half the exposure of venlafaxine, with no adverse effects reported in breastfed infants (Kronenfeld et al., 2017). Milk levels for both duloxetine and reboxetine are low, with no adverse effects reported in breastfed infants (Kronenfeld et al., 2017).

As for other types of antidepressants, bupropion levels are low in milk. However, concerns about seizures have been raised. It also has an active metabolite (Kronenfeld et al., 2017). Unfortunately, this medication is often suggested for the condition known as D-MER (dysphoric milk-ejection reflex) (Heise & Wiessinger, 2011), even though no studies have demonstrated its efficacy.

Clinical Takeaways

- Antidepressants can be used during pregnancy, but they can lead to complications such as preterm birth. Children may also have some cognitive and behavioral effects, but those appear to be transitory. Generally speaking, many clinicians feel that the benefits of antidepressants outweigh the risks associated with untreated depression.
- However, given the large number of non-drug treatments that work as well as medications, other clinicians prefer them.
- Some antidepressants have very low transfer rates into breastmilk. These can be safer choices to prescribe (e.g., sertraline and paroxetine).
- One longitudinal study revealed that approximately 50% of mothers who were treated with antidepressants during pregnancy were still depressed at 4 years postpartum. This study highlights why continuous assessment is important.

21 Atypical Antidepressants
Ketamine and Brexanolone

There are two newer options for treating severe depression. Ketamine and brexanolone produce rapid results and treat severe depression and suicidal ideation. Rather than change levels of serotonin-norepinephrine and dopamine, as typical antidepressants do, these medications work on the neurotransmitters GABA (γ-aminobutyric acid) and glutamate.

KEY FINDINGS

- Ketamine and brexanolone treat depression quickly and are delivered via IV infusion.
- Esketamine is an iteration of ketamine that uses only the S isomer. It can be delivered intranasally and is FDA-approved as a "breakthrough" treatment for depression.
- Brexanolone was designed specifically to treat postpartum depression and has been FDA-approved for that purpose. However, its cost is extremely high and may not be as accessible as esketamine.

GABA and Glutamate

GABA is an inhibitory neurotransmitter; it calms the brain and lessens nerves' ability to create, send, or receive chemical messages. When nerves are hyperactive, they increase symptoms of anxiety, stress, and fear. In contrast, glutamate is an excitatory neurotransmitter. Health require that GABA and glutamate be balanced. When GABA and glutamate are out of balance, depression and other neuropsychiatric conditions are also more likely (Jia-Hui et al., 2019). Women with postpartum depression had altered glutamate concentrations in the dorsolateral prefrontal cortex, a pattern seen in other types of depression (Jia-Hui et al., 2019). Stress is the primary risk factor for depression, and glutamate underlies HPA axis activity induced by chronic stress.

N-methyl-D-aspartate (NMDA) is a glutamate receptor. There are NMDA receptors in the hippocampus, which is crucial to memory development. NMDA affects the lifelong development of the brain. NMDA receptors are also involved in excitotoxicity, which plays a role in diseases such as epilepsy or Alzheimer's. Many drugs inhibit NMDA receptors, including drugs of abuse (such as ketamine). To be most effective, NMDA antagonists need to block excessive activation without interfering with normal functioning. GABA receptors (particularly $GABA_B$ receptors) affect the expression, signaling, and activity of the glutamate receptors. Conversely, NMDA receptors affect $GABA_B$ expression and function (Kantamneni, 2015).

DOI: 10.4324/9781003405092-26

Glutamate and NMDA receptors are also potentially involved in fear conditioning and the pathophysiology of PTSD (Kelmendi et al., 2017). Glutamatergic projections from the prefrontal cortex, hippocampus, and amygdala modulate fear learning, extinction learning, and contextual fear conditioning. Medications that can block memory consolidation after a traumatic event lessen PTSD. However, using it too soon after a traumatic event can cause dissociation, which makes PTSD more likely.

Luscher and Mohler (2019) argue that chronic stress impairs GABAergic inhibition and increases glutamate release, which chronically dysregulates the stress axis and increases the risk for anxiety and major depression. Conversely, GABAergic inhibition increases stress resilience. Both ketamine and brexanolone affect GABA and glutamate, but in different ways. Brexanolone restores and super-potentiates GABAergic neural inhibition that allows glutamate receptors to rapidly recover cell surface expression, which normalizes synaptic function and recovery of normal neural connectivity. Ketamine briefly inhibits GABAergic interneurons, followed by a transient surge in glutamate release that triggers the release of brain-derived neurotrophic factor (BDNF) and a wave of synaptic genesis. Both new medications offer rapid relief from severe depression and are important parts of the treatment arsenal.

Ketamine

Ketamine is an anesthetic medication with an off-label use to treat severe refractory depression, especially depression with suicide risk (Preston et al., 2022). Around 60% of patients respond 4.5 hours after a single dose, which lasts 24 hours. The response rate is over 40% after 7 days (Molero et al., 2018). Repeated doses (2 to 4 times per week) sustain the response for several weeks. Ketamine is administered in a clinic via IV over a 2- to 3-hour period, with healthcare providers monitoring for possible dissociative and psychotic (temporary) symptoms. There is also an intranasal version: esketamine (see next section).

Ketamine is an antagonist of NMDA receptors and blocks their activity. It is available in two forms: racemic ketamine and S-ketamine. Racemic ketamine contains S- and R-isomers, which mirror each other. IV ketamine infusions use both S- and R-ketamine. In their review of 3 randomized trials, 8 open-label trials, and 30 case reports, Smith-Apeldoorn and colleagues (2022) noted that ketamine has been administered intravenously, intranasally, orally, and possibly intramuscularly. Side effects were uncommon but included possible elevated blood pressure and mild dissociative and psychotomimetic effects. They concluded that ketamine had "therapeutic potential" (p. 907) and that maintenance ketamine treatment sustains its antidepressant effect.

Another review and meta-analysis of 24 trials ($N = 1,877$) compared the efficacy of racemic vs. esketamine for depression and bipolar major depression (Bahji et al., 2021). Racemic ketamine produced a greater treatment response, higher remission rates, and lower dropouts due to adverse effects compared to esketamine. Some participants were also using psychotropic medications or receiving psychotherapy. The authors noted that proof of efficacy remains low and encouraged futured clinical trials. Ketamine works quickly and lowers depression with suicidal ideations so could be effective for some high-risk mothers.

Esketamine

Esketamine (Spravato) is a recent iteration that uses only the S-isomer. The US Food and Drug Administration (FDA) approved esketamine to treat depression and lower suicide risk on March 5, 2019. Intranasal esketamine was comparable to IV infusions in its antidepressant effect, and the FDA designated it a "breakthrough therapy" (Molero et al., 2018). Esketamine is a glutamate NMDA antagonist, but its specific mechanism vis-à-vis depression is unknown. Effects are seen within minutes to hours.

A recent phase-2, double-blind, randomized placebo-controlled trial compared esketamine in three different dosages (28, 56, and 84 milligrams) to a placebo administered twice a week (Daly et al., 2018). The final sample included 67 participants with treatment-resistant major depression that had not responded to two or more antidepressants. They continued taking their medications during the trial. Esketamine was superior to the placebo in all three groups, and symptom improvement was sustained despite reduced frequency of use. The results persisted for more than 2 months.

An expert opinion article noted that ketamine produced rapid antidepressant effects (Nikayin et al., 2022). Regarding safety for racemic ketamine and esketamine, they noted that high-dose ketamine can cause long-term cognitive impairment, but esketamine did not have these effects, with no increased risk for cognitive impairment, when used appropriately. Another expert opinion stated that:

> Intranasal esketamine is a new treatment option for people with TRD [treatment-resistant depression]. The main benefit of esketamine is rapid onset of antidepressant activity, but effects of prolonged treatment are still preliminary. The main concerns relate to the safety aspects of prolonged esketamine therapy when considering its abuse potential. While data for esketamine use over a long period of time is lacking, its use should be carefully monitored.
>
> (Kryst et al., 2020, p. 9).

Questions remain, however, regarding how to maintain ketamine's antidepressant effect after acute administration and the safety of ketamine and esketamine long-term. Specific concerns are neurocognitive and urologic toxicity, and possible addiction (Molero et al., 2018).

Ketamine Use in Postpartum Women

To date, ketamine has not been used to treat postpartum depression. Much of the postpartum research on ketamine comes from China. The studies used ketamine to prevent depression in women who had cesarean sections (Zhang, Betran, et al., 2022). For example, a Chinese randomized, controlled, double-blind study gave 327 women ketamine immediately post-op, while another 327 received a placebo and usual care (Jia-Hui et al., 2019). Women in the ketamine group had lower scores on the EPDS at 4 days and 42 days compared to the placebo group. The prevalence of depression in the ketamine group was 13% and 20% in the control group. Ketamine also lowered suicidal ideation and incidence of the blues. There were some side effects in the intervention group: 19% vomited, and 4 women hallucinated. However, these symptoms were transient (Jia-Hui et al., 2019).

Another study from Iran had a similar design (Alipoor et al., 2021). One hundred and thirty-four women who had planned cesareans were randomized to receive Nesdonal (thiopental) as an anesthesia with (intervention) or without (control) ketamine. They measured depression before the cesarean, and at 2 and 4 weeks after. The women who received ketamine were significantly less depressed at 4 weeks. However, all the mothers were significantly depressed before they had their cesareans (with a score of 13 or higher on the EDPS). The best result was when depression dropped to 10 on the EPDS at 4 weeks, which is still depressed. This is an improvement, but ketamine during a cesarean did not lead to remission. Further, what they did not say, but was true, based on the medications that they reported, is that these mothers had planned cesareans *under general anesthesia*, which makes their experience more severe.

Brexanolone

Brexanolone is a medication specifically designed to treat postpartum depression and received FDA approval for that in 2019. It is a synthetic version of allopregnanolone, a neurosteroid and metabolite of progesterone that acts on GABA receptors (Walkery et al., 2021). Specifically, $GABA_A$ agonists slow the recovery of the $GABA_A$ receptor from desensitization. Allopregnanolone modulates the strength of the $GABA_A$ receptors, the mechanism by which it regulates emotional behavior. SSRIs have a similar mechanism (Griffin & Mellon, 1999).

Brexanolone rapidly treats depression, with a fast drop in symptoms and remission that is sustained for at least 30 days. Sage Therapeutics, maker of brexanolone, notes that SSRIs were designed to treat depression in general but do not reduce symptoms for at least 6 weeks. Sage Therapeutics noted that patients on SSRIs are often undermedicated, may stop taking their medications because of side effects, or may experience withdrawal symptoms if they stop. In addition, clinicians often do not provide adequate follow-up. For these reasons, they feel that their product is superior to SSRIs. They concede that cost and side effects, such as loss of consciousness, remain "sizeable obstacles" that will need to be overcome (Gerbasi et al., 2021). However, they still consider brexanolone a cost-effective option if considered over an 11-year period compared with treating someone with SSRIs for the same amount of time.

Although allopregnanolone seems like a new approach, the theory behind it has been around for a long time. Progesterone, along with allopregnanolone, drops precipitously postpartum. An allopregnanolone agonist is used to increase the amount of available allopregnanolone, which is a similar model to studies that used progesterone to decrease depression. One recent article that described brexanolone explicitly referenced this theory but added the twist of their impact on GABA receptors.

> Researchers have postulated that rapid alternations in the concentration of neuroactive steroids, such as allopregnanolone, during the peripartum period may contribute to affective dysregulation in women. Allopregnanolone rises with progesterone throughout pregnancy and peaks in the third trimester. Allopregnanolone is a modulator of γ-aminobutyric acid-A (GABA-A) receptors, and if these receptors do not adjust to the fluctuations in hormone levels after birth, this may be one mechanism that contributes to the development of PPD.
>
> (Fantasia, 2019, p. 451)

Another recent review made a similar connection between hormonal shifts and postpartum depression.

> The peripartum period is characterized by rapid and significant physiological change in plasma levels of endocrine hormones, peptides, and neuroactive steroids.

Evidence supporting the role of neuroactive steroids and GABA in the pathophysiology of postpartum depression led to the investigation of synthetic neuroactive steroids and their analogs as potential treatment for postpartum depression. Brexanolone, a soluble, proprietary, intravenous preparation of synthetic allopregnanolone has been developed.

Walkery et al. (2021) noted that while the unique mechanism is not fully understood, the hypothesis is that an allopregnanolone agonists restore allopregnanolone concentrations and reset neural networks, which improves postpartum depression symptoms. Allopregnanolone also reduces inflammation, which is another proposed mechanism for its efficacy (Cornett et al., 2021).

Efficacy

A recent review described three studies that tested the efficacy and safety of brexanolone in treating postpartum depression. One study was a phase II trial, and the others were phase III. None of the mothers were breastfeeding. Two-thirds were Black in the initial trial, and some were also taking antidepressants. The sample sizes were small ($N = 4$ in the treatment group and $N = 8$ in the placebo group). The second study included 138 women randomized into three treatment groups (two different dosages of brexanolone or a placebo). Two-thirds of these women were White. The depression scores at the end of the infusion were significantly lower, and a higher percentage achieved remission compared to the placebo group.

The third trial included 108 patients: 54 received brexanolone, and 54 received the placebo. The remission rates were higher in the treatment group, but the effect was not maintained at follow-up. In all three studies, brexanolone was not superior to the placebo at 30 days (Walkery et al., 2021). Two authors disclosed financial connections to pharmaceutical companies, including the manufacturer of brexanolone.

A recent analysis pooled data from previously published phase 2 and phase 3 data and conducted post hoc analyses. The sample included 209 patients who received either brexanolone or a placebo. The authors reported meaningful clinical changes after the 60-hour treatment, with a more rapid decline in symptoms in the treatment group and sustained improvements. In the treatment group, there was a significantly higher percentage of clinical responders and remitters, based on their scores from the Hamilton Depression Rating Scale (HAM-D) (Gerbasi et al., 2021). Several of the authors are employees of Sage Therapeutics, and most have a financial stake in the company. Two authors were paid by Sage to conduct this research.

A recent network meta-analysis compared efficacy of brexanolone injections with SSRIs for treating postpartum depression (Cooper et al., 2019). They identified 26 studies and found 6 with the same design: brexanolone vs. placebo and SSRIs vs. placebo at day 3, week 4, and last observation. They calculated change from baseline based on results from the EPDS and the HAM-D. At all time points, change from baseline was greater for brexanolone than for SSRIs, but the difference between the two treatments was less at every assessment point on both scales. SSRIs do not become effective until 4 to 6 weeks after administration. Brexanolone treats symptoms more quickly than SSRIs (as it is designed to do) but is not necessarily better than SSRIs over the long term. In cases of severe depression, both could be used: brexanolone to address immediate symptoms, and SSRIs to maintain recovery.

Limitations of Brexanolone

Brexanolone has been heavily marketed to practitioners and "influencers" in the postpartum depression field (including me). Many were excited about a depression treatment that targeted GABA receptors, feeling that this was a "new" model of treatment that reverses depression quickly. However, in some ways, it is not new at all. Allopregnanolone is a metabolite of progesterone, which has a long, and now discredited, use as a treatment, and mutes my enthusiasm. There are also some significant practical downsides.

Brexanolone requires IV infusion over 60 hours and must be administered in the hospital (Walkery et al., 2021) because of its black box warning for "potential excessive sedation and sudden loss of consciousness" (p. 451) (Fantasia, 2019). Approximately 30% of women experience a significant drop in symptoms that last at least a month. But most patients are co-treated with other antidepressants. The cost of the medication is significant (approximately $34,000 plus fees for the hospital stay and for clinician care). It also involves being separated from infants during that time. Finally, breastfeeding women were specifically excluded from trials, possibly because a progesterone metabolite might cause breastfeeding to fail. Progesterone specifically blocks the hormone prolactin. This is why progesterone levels naturally plummet postpartum.

Cornett and colleagues (2021) also noted that brexanolone requires hospitalization, IV administration, and high costs. It also carries the risk of sedation or loss of consciousness. I would add separation of mothers from their newborns for 60 hours and inability to breastfeed. Some may be offered this treatment, as they were offered estrogen patches or progesterone suppositories in earlier times, without realizing its negative effects on breastfeeding and/or mother-infant separation.

Zuranolone

A variant of brexanolone, zuranolone, may address some of these concerns. Zuranolone also treats depressive symptoms via the GABA receptors. It has a similar mechanism of action and pharmacokinetic profile for brexanolone but is administered orally once a day. In a randomized trial, 150 patients with depression received either a placebo or 30 mg of zuranolone (Deligiannidis et al., 2021). Patients receiving zuranolone had lower symptoms by Day 3, which is unusual for an antidepressant. By Day 15, patients in the zuranolone group had significantly lower scores on the Hamilton Depression Rating Scale. The effect was sustained through Day 45. These findings are promising.

Clinical Takeaways

- Brexanolone and esketamine are important additions for treating severe depression. They are preferable to electroconvulsive therapy (ECT), which is sometimes used to treat severe refractory depression.
- Brexanolone and esketamine can be used with typical antidepressants. Brexanolone and esketamine quickly reduce symptoms, while antidepressants maintain the effect.
- Esketamine will likely be more accessible to mothers, especially since it can be delivered intranasally. Brexanolone requires 60 hours of hospitalization to administer. The medication alone may also be prohibitively expensive.
  Esketamine can become a drug of abuse, so clinicians must carefully administer it.
- Zuranolone may overcome the challenges inherent in using brexanolone.

22 Putting It All Together

In this final chapter, I offer some practical suggestions for synthesizing information in this book and taking the next steps. You may be setting up or adding to your program. You can decide how to and where to screen, and which interventions are feasible for your community. Telehealth has also increased access to specialized care for many smaller and rural communities. Here is one way to think through the next steps.

1. **Select your screening tool.** This is the first step. Which tool will you select? How will it be distributed? Will it go to every mother (recommended) or only ones who have symptoms? Will the screening tool be paper or electronic? If you are using the EPDS, which cutoff will you use? Will it be a wide or more narrow screen? Who will collect and score the information? How will mothers who screen positive be contacted?
2. **Establish baseline health.** I recommend checking on the physical health for all your mothers. If that is not possible for everyone, prioritize those who screened positive. I recommend checking vitamins D and B-12 to ensure that mothers are not deficient. I would also recommend that mothers be checked for hypothyroidism (T3, T4, TSH), anemia, and possible inflammation (complete blood count and C-reactive protein).
3. **Consider anti-inflammatory supplements (EPA and curcumin).** Lowering inflammation is an important part of recovering from depression. If mothers are open to it, you might suggest that they supplement with 1,000 milligrams of EPA and 500 milligrams of curcumin twice a day. This will be good for their physical and mental health.
4. **Will you treat or refer?** Thinking through your scope of practice, what areas can you address? Could you set up a peer or professional support network in your community (or is one already available)? Who will be in your referral network? Have you talked to them about seeing some of your clients?
5. **Identify the treatments that mothers can access in your community.** Consider exercise, bright light therapy, acupuncture, transcranial magnetic stimulation, or medications. What types of psychotherapy are available? Could mothers access these? What telehealth options are available?
6. **Evaluate your efforts.** Many therapies take 4 to 6 weeks to be effective. When will you reassess mothers to see how they are doing? Many programs never check, but it is important that you do. No treatment works for everyone—even medications. The goal is for mothers' symptoms to remit. Assessment can stop once mothers are better.

DOI: 10.4324/9781003405092-27

I am excited for you to put this information to use. Even small efforts will help. The work you are doing has long-term implications. New mothers' mental health influences everyone in their families. Your efforts will have an impact far beyond the perinatal period.

Thank you for your willingness to stand in the gap for new mothers and their families. The difference you make will last for years.

References

Abdel-Salam, O. M. (2005). Anti-inflammatory, antinociceptive, and gastric effects of Hypericum perforatum in rats. *Scientific World Journal, 5*, 586–595.

Abdollahpour, S., Khosravi, A., & Bolbolhaghighi, N. (2016). The effect of the magical hour on post-traumatic stress disorder (PTSD) in traumatic childbirth: A clinical trial. *Journal of Reproductive and Infant Psychology, 34*(4), 403–412. https://doi.org/10.1080/02646838.2016.1185773

Academy of Breastfeeding Medicine. (2008). ABM clinical protocol #6: Guideline on co-sleeping and breastfeeding. *Breastfeeding Medicine, 3*(1), 38–43.

Afand, N., Keshavarz, M., Fatemi, N. S., & Montazeri, A. (2016). Effects of infant massage on state anxiety in mothers of preterm infants prior to hospital discharge. *Journal of Clinical Nursing, 26*, 1887–1892. https://doi.org/10.1111/jocn.13498

Afshariani, R., Farhadi, P., Ghaffarpasand, F., & Roozbeh, J. (2014). Effectiveness of topical curcumin for treatment of mastitis in breastfeeding women: A randomized, double-blind, placebo-controlled clinical trial. *Oman Medical Journal, 29*(5), 330–334. https://doi.org/10.5001/omj.2014.89

Alder, J., Stadlmayr, W., Tschudin, S., & Bitzer, J. (2006). Post-traumatic symptoms after childbirth: What should we offer? *Journal of Psychosomatic Obstetrics & Gynecology, 27*(2), 107–112.

Alipoor, M., Loripoor, M., Kazemi, M., Farahbakhsh, F., & Sarkoohi, A. (2021). The effect of ketamine on preventing postpartum depression. *Journal of Medicine and Life, 41*(1), 87–92. https://doi.org/10.25122/jml-2020-0116

Amani, B., Merza, D., Savoy, C., Streiner, D., Bieling, P., Ferro, M. A., & Van Lieshout, R. J. (2022). Peer-delivered cognitive-behavioral therapy for postpartum depression: A randomized controlled trial. *Journal of Clinical Psychiatry, 83*(1). https://doi.org/10.4088/JCP.21m13928

American College of Obstetricians and Gynecologists. (2015). The American College of Obstetricians and Gynecologists Committee Opinion No. 630 screening for perinatal depression. *Obstetrics & Gynecology, 125*, 1268–1271.

American College of Obstetricians and Gynecologists. (2023, June). *Treatment and management of mental health conditions during pregnancy and postpartum, 5.* www.acog.org/clinical/clinical-guidance/clinical-practice-guideline/articles/2023/06/treatment-and-management-of-mental-health-conditions-during-pregnancy-and-postpartum

American Psychological Association. (2017). *Clinical practice guidelines for the treatment of post-traumatic stress disorder.* www.apa.org/ptsd-guideline/treatments/cognitive-therapy

Amini, S., Jafarirad, S., & Amani, R. (2019). Postpartum depression and vitamin D: A systematic review. *Critical Reviews in Food Science and Nutrition, 59*(9), 1514–1520. https://doi.org/10.1080/10408398.2017.1423276

Amorin, A. R., Linne, Y. M., & Lourenco, P. M. (2007, July 18). Diet or exercise, or both, for weight reduction in women after childbirth. *Cochrane Database Systematic Review.* https://doi.org/CD005627

Angelotta, C., & Wisner, K. L. (2017). Treating depression during pregnancy: Are we asking the right questions? *Birth Defects Research, 109*, 879–887. https://doi.org/10.1002/bdr2.1074

Anghelescu, I. G., Kohnen, R., Szegedi, A., Klement, S., & Kieser, M. (2006). Comparison of Hypericum extract WS 5570 and paroxetine in ongoing treatment after recovery from an episode of moderate to severe depression: Results from a randomized multicenter study. *Pharmacopsychiatry, 39*, 213–219.

Appels, A., Golombeck, B., Gorgels, A., de Vreede, J., & van Bruekelen, G. (2000). Behavioral risk factors of sudden cardiac arrest. *Journal of Psychosomatic Research, 48*, 463–469.

Arch, J. J., Dimidjian, S., & Chessick, C. (2012). Are exposure-based cognitive-behavioral therapies safe during pregnancy. *Archives of Women's Mental Health, 15*, 445–457.

Ayers, S., Wright, D. B., & Thornton, A. (2018). Development of a measure of postpartum PTSD: The City Birth Trauma Scale. *Frontiers in Psychiatry, 9*.

Babyak, M., Blumenthal, J. A., Herman, S., Khatri, P., Doraiswamy, M., Moore, K., Craighead, W. E., Baldewicz, T. T., & Krishnan, R. R. (2000). Exercise treatment for major depression: Maintenance of therapeutic benefit at 10 months. *Psychosomatic Medicine, 62*, 633–638.

Bahji, A., Vazquez, G. H., & Zarate, C. A. (2021). Comparative efficacy of racemic ketamine and esketamine for depression: A systematic review and meta-analysis. *Journal of Affective Disorders, 278*, 542–555. https://doi.org/10.1016/j.jad.2020.09.071

Bai, D. L., Wu, K. M., & Tarrant, M. (2013). Association between intrapartum interventions and breastfeeding duration. *Journal of Midwifery and Women's Health, 58*(1), 25–32. https://doi.org/10.1111/j.1542-2011.2012.00254.x

Bais, B., Kamperman, A. M., Bijma, H. H., Hoogendijk, W. J., Souman, J. L., Knijff, E., & Lambregtse-van den Berg, M. P. (2020). Effects of bright light therapy for depression during pregnancy: A randomised, double-blind controlled trial. *BMJ Open, 10*(10). https://doi.org/10.1136/bmjopen-2020-038030

Ball, H. L., Moya, E., Fairley, L., Westman, J., Oddie, S., & Wright, J. (2012). Infant care practices related to sudden infant death syndrome in South Asian and white British families in the UK. *Paediatric and Perinatal Epidemiology, 26*, 3–12.

Barrera, A., Moh, Y. S., Nichols, A., & Le, H.-N. (2021). The factor reliability and convergent validity of the Patient Health Questionnaire-4 among an international sample of pregnant women. *Journal of Women's Health (Larchmont), 30*(4), 525–532. https://doi.org/10.1089/jwh.2020.8320

Barsaglini, A., Sartori, G., Benetti, S., Pettersson-Yeo, W., & Mechelli, A. (2014). The effects of psychotherapy on brain function: A systematic and critical review. *Progress in Neurobiology, 114*, 1–14.

Basu, A., Kim, H. H., Basaldua, R., Choi, K. W., Charron, L., Kelsall, N., Hernandez-Diaz, S., Wyszynski, D. F., & Koenen, K. C. (2021). A cross-national study of factors associated with women's perinatal mental health and wellbeing during the COVID-19 pandemic. *PLoS One, 16*(4). https://doi.org/10.1371/journal.pone.0249780

Beck, C. T., & Gable, R. K. (2000). Postpartum Depression Screening Scale: Development and psychometric testing. *Nursing Research, 49*, 155–164.

Belleville, G., Guay, S., & Marchand, A. (2011). Persistence of sleep disturbances following cognitive-behavioral therapy for posttraumatic stress disorder. *Journal of Psychosomatic Research, 70*, 318–327.

Berk, M., Williams, L. J., Jacka, F. N., O'Neil, A., Pasco, J. A., Moylan, S., Allen, N. B., Stuart, A. L., Hayley, A. C., Byrne, M. L., & Maes, M. (2013). So depression is an inflammatory disease, but where does the inflammation come from? *BMC Medicine, 11*, 200. www.biomedcentral.com/1741-7015/11/200

Bigelow, A., Power, M., MacLellan-Peters, J., Alex, M., & McDonald, C. (2012). Effect of mother/infant skin-to-skin contact on postpartum depressive symptoms and maternal physiological stress. *Journal of Obstetric, Gynecologic, and Neonatal Nursing, 41*, 369–382.

Bilszta, J. L. C., Tsuchiya, S., Han, K., Buist, A., & Einarson, A. (2011). Primary care physician's attitudes and practices regarding antidepressants use during pregnancy: A survey of two countries. *Archives of Women's Mental Health, 14*, 71–75.

Bina, R. (2020). Predictors of postpartum depression service use: A theory-informed, integrative systematic review. *Women & Birth, 33*, e24–e32. https://doi.org/10.1016/j.wombi.2019.01.006

Blevins, C. A., Weathers, F. W., Davis, M. T., Witte, T. K., & Domino, J. L. (2015). The Posttraumatic Stress Disorder Checklist for DSM-5 (PCL-5): Development and initial psychometric evaluation. *Journal of Traumatic Stress, 28*(6), 489–498. https://doi.org/10.1002/jts.22059

Blumenthal, J. A., Babyak, M. A., Doraiswamy, P. M., Watkins, L., Hoffman, B. M., Barbour, K. A., Herman, S., Edward Craighead, W., Brosse, A. L., Waugh, R., Hinderliter, A., and Sherwood, A. (2007). Exercise and pharmacotherapy in the treatment of major depressive disorder. *Psychosomatic Medicine, 69*, 587–596.

Bluth, K., & Blanton, P. W. (2014). Mindfulness and self-compassion: Exploring pathways to adolescent emotional well-being. *Journal of Child Family Studies, 23*(7), 1298–1309. https://doi.org/10.1007/s10826-013-9830-2

Bobo, W. V., Epstein, R. A., Hayes, R. M., Shelton, R. C., Hartert, T. V., Mitchel, E., Horner, J., & Wu, P. (2014). The effect of regulatory advisories on maternal antidepressant prescriptions, 1995–2007: An interrupted time series study on 228,876 pregnancies. *Archives of Women's Mental Health, 17*, 17–26.

Boyce, P., & Condon, J. (2001). Providing good clinical care means listening to women's concerns. *British Medical Journal, 322*, 928.

Brandon, A. R., Ceccotti, N., Hynan, L. S., Shivakumar, G., Johnson, N., & Jarrett, R. B. (2012). Proof of concept: Partner-assisted interpersonal psychotherapy for perinatal depression. *Archives of Women's Mental Health, 15*, 469–480.

Bratman, S., & Girman, A. M. (2003). *Handbook of herbs and supplements and their therapeutic uses.* Mosby.

Burns, D. (1999). *Feeling good: The new mood therapy.* William Morrow.

Buttner, M. M., Brock, R. L., O'Hara, M. W., & Stuart, S. (2015). Efficacy of yoga for depressed postpartum women: A randomized controlled trial. *Complementary Therapies in Clinical Practice, 21*(2), 94–100. https://doi.org/10.1016/j.ctcp.2015.03.003

Buysse, D. J., Reynolds, C. F., Monk, T. H., Berman, S. R., & Kupfer, D. (1989). The Pittsburgh Sleep Quality Index: A new instrument for psychiatric practice and research. *Psychiatric Research, 28*(2), 193–213. https://doi.org/10.1016/0165-1781(89)90047-4

Byatt, N., Biebel, K., Friedman, L., Debordes-Jackson, G., & Ziedonis, D. (2013). Women's perspectives on postpartum depression screening in pediatric settings. *Archives of Women's Mental Health, 16*, 429–432.

Caparros-Gonzalez, R. A., Romero-Gonzalez, B., Peralta-Ramirez, M. I., Galan-Paredes, A., & Caracuel-Romero, A. (2021). Assessment of posttraumatic stress disorder among women after childbirth using the City Birth Trauma Scale in Spain. *Psychological Trauma, 13*(5), 545–554. https://doi.org/10.1037/tra0001007

Cappelletti, M., Della Bella, S., Ferrazzi, E., Mavilio, D., & Divanovic, S. (2016). Inflammation and preterm birth. *Journal of Leukocyte Biology, 99*, 67–78. https://doi.org/10.1189/jlb.3MR0615-272RR

Carter, T., Bastounis, A., Guo, B., & Morrell, C. J. (2019). The effectiveness of exercise-based interventions for preventing or treating postpartum depression: A systematic review and meta-analysis. *Archives of Women's Mental Health, 22*, 37–53. https://doi.org/10.1007/s00737-018-0869-3

Centers for Disease Control. (2019). *Infant mortality.* www.cdc.gov/reproductivehealth/maternal-infanthealth/infantmortality.htm

Chabrol, H., & Teissedre, J. (2004). Relation between Edinburgh Postnatal Depression Scale scores at 2–3 days and 4–6 weeks postpartum. *Journal of Reproductive and Infant Psychology, 22*(1), 33–39.

Chabrol, H., Teissedre, J., Armitage, M. D., & Walburg, V. (2004). Acceptability of psychotherapy and antidepressants for postnatal depression among newly delivered mothers. *Journal of Reproductive and Infant Psychology, 22*(1), 5–12.

Chaudron, L. H. (2007). Treating pregnant women with antidepressants: The gray zone. *Journal of Women's Health, 16*(4), 551–553.

Cheng, B., Roberts, N., Wang, X., Li, Y., Chen, Y., Zhao, Y., Deng, P., Meng, Y., Deng, W., & Wang, J. (2022). Social support mediates the influence of cerebellum functional connectivity strength on postpartum depression and postpartum depression with anxiety. *Translational Psychiatry, 12*. https://doi.org/10.1038/s41398-022-01781-9

Cho, H. J., Kwon, J. H., & Lee, J. J. (2008). Antenatal cognitive-behavioral therapy for prevention of postpartum depression: A pilot study. *Yonsei Medical Journal, 49*(4), 553–562.

Chong, M. F. F., Ong, Y.-L., Calder, P. C., Colega, M., Wong, J. X. Y., Tan, C. S., & Lim, A. L. (2015). Long-chain polyunsaturated fatty acid status during pregnancy and maternal mental health in pregnancy and the postpartum period: Results from the GUSTO study. *Journal of Clinical Psychiatry, 76*, e848–e856.

Ciappolino, V., Delvecchio, G., Agostoni, C., Mazzocchi, A., Altamura, A. C., & Brambillo, P. (2017). The role of n-3 polyunsaturated fatty acids (n-3 PUFAs) in affective disorders. *Journal of Affective Disorders, 224*, 32–47.

Claridge, A. M. (2014). Efficacy of systemically oriented psychotherapies in the treatment of perinatal depression: A meta-analysis. *Archives of Women's Mental Health, 17*, 3–15.

Clark, C. T., & Wisner, K. L. (2018). Treatment of peripartum bipolar disorder. *Obstetric & Gynecology Clinics of North America, 45*, 403–417. https://doi.org/10.1016/j.ogc.2018.05.002

Cooney, G. M., Dwan, K., Grieg, C. A., Lawlor, D. A., Rimer, J., Waugh, F. R., McMurdo, M., & Mead, G. E. (2013). Exercise for depression. *Cochrane Database of Systematic Reviews, 12*, https://doi.org/10.1002/14651858.CD004366.pu66

Cooper, M. C., Kilvert, H. S., Hodgkins, P., Roskell, N. S., & Eldar-Lissai, A. (2019). Using matching-adjusted indirect comparisons and network meta-analyses to compare efficacy of brexanolone injection with selective-serotonin reuptake inhibitors for treating postpartum depression. *CNS Drugs, 33*(10), 1039–1052. https://doi.org/10.1007/s40263-019-00672-w

Cooper, P. J., Landman, M., Tomlinson, M., Molteno, C., Swartz, L., & Murray, L. (2002). *British Journal of Psychiatry, 180*, 76–81.

Cooper, P. J., Landman, M., Tomlinson, M., Molteno, C., Swartz, L., & Murray, L. (2002). Impact of a mother-infant intervention in an indigent peri-urban South African context: Pilot study. *British Journal of Psychiatry, 180*, 76–81.

Cornett, E. M., Rando, L., Labbe, A. M., Perkins, W., Kaye, A. M., Kaye, A. D., Viswanath, O., & Urits, I. (2021). Brexanolone to treat postpartum depression in adult women. *Psychopharmacology Bulletin, 51*(2), 115–130.

Corral, M., Kuan, A., & Kostaras, D. (2000). Bright light therapy's effect on postpartum depression. *American Journal of Psychiatry, 157*, 303–304.

Coussons-Read, M. E., Lobel, M., Carey, J. C., Kreither, M. O., D'Anna, K., Argys, L., Ross, R. G., Brandt, C., & Cole, S. (2012). The occurrence of preterm delivery is linked to pregnancy-specific distress and elevated inflammatory markers across gestation. *Brain, Behavior & Immunity, 26*, 650–659.

Coussons-Read, M. E., Okun, M. L., Schmitt, M. P., & Giese, S. (2005). Prenatal stress alters cytokine levels in a manner that may endanger human pregnancy. *Psychosomatic Medicine, 67*, 625–631.

Cox, E. Q., Killenberg, S., Frische, R., McClure, R., Hill, M., Jenson, J., Pearson, B., & Meltzer-Brody, S. (2020). Repetitive transcranial magnetic stimulation for the treatment of postpartum depression. *Journal of Affective Disorders, 264*, 193–200. https://doi.org/10.1016/j.jad.2019.11.069

Cox, J. (2019). Thirty years with the Edinburgh Postnatal Depression Scale: Voices from the past and recommendations for the future. *British Journal of Psychiatry, 214*, 127–129. https://doi.org/10.1192/bjp.2018.245

Cox, J. L., Holden, J. M., & Sagovsky, R. (1987). Detection of postnatal depression: Development of the 10-item Edinburgh Postnatal Depression Scale. *British Journal of Psychiatry, 150*, 782–786.

Crawley, R., Ayers, S., Button, S., Thornton, A., Field, A. P., Lee, S., Eagle, A., Bradley, R., Moore, D., Gyte, G., & Smith, H. (2018). Feasibility and acceptability of expressive writing with postpartum women: A randomised controlled trial. *BMC Pregnancy and Childbirth, 18*(75). https://doi.org/10.1186/s12884-018-1703-7

Crowley, S. K., & Youngstedt, S. D. (2012). Efficacy of light therapy for perinatal depression: A review. *Journal of Physiological Anthropology, 31*, 15.

Currie, M. L., & Rademacher, R. (2004). The pediatrician's role in recognizing and intervening in postpartum depression. *Pediatric Clinics of North America, 51*, 785–801.

Cutler, C. B., Legano, L. A., Dreyer, B. P., Fierman, A. H., Berkule, S. B., Lusskin, S. I., Tomopoulos, S., Roth, M., & Mendelsohn, A. L. (2007). Screening for maternal depression in a low education population using a two-item questionnaire. *Archives of Women's Mental Health, 10*, 277–283.

Daley, A. J., Foster, L., Long, G., Palmer, C., Robinson, O., Walmsley, H., & Ward, R. M. (2015). The effectiveness of exercise for the prevention and treatment of antenatal depression: A systematic review with meta-analysis. *British Journal of Obstetrics & Gynaecology, 58*, 178–183.

Daley, A. J., Macarthur, C., & Winter, H. (2007). The role of exercise in treating postpartum depression: A review of the literature. *Journal of Midwifery and Women's Health, 52*, 56–62.

Daley, A. J., Winter, H., Grimmett, C., McGuinness, M., McManus, R., & MacArthur, C. (2008). Feasibility of an exercise intervention for women with postnatal depression: A pilot randomised controlled trial. *British Journal of General Practice, 58*, 178–183.

Daly, E. J., Singh, J. B., Fedgchin, M., Cooper, K., Lim, P., Shelton, R. C., Thase, M. E., Winokur, A., Van Nueten, L., Manji, H., & Drevets, W. C. (2018). Efficacy and safety of intranasal esketamine adjunctive to oral antidepressant therapy in a treatment-resistant depression: A randomized clinical trial. *JAMA Psychiatry, 75*(2), 139–148. https://doi.org/10.1001/jamapsychiatry.2017.3739

Davenport, M. H., McCurdy, A. P., Mottola, M. F., Skow, R. J., Meah, V. L., & Poitras, V. J. (2018). Impact of prenatal exercise on both prenatal and postnatal anxiety and depressive symptoms: A systematic review and meta-analysis. *British Journal of Sports Medicine, 52*, 1376–1385. https://doi.org/10.1136bjsports-2018-099697

Davidson, E. L., & Ollerton, R. L. (2020). Partners behaviours improving breastfeeding outcomes: An integrative review. *Women & Birth, 33*(1), e15–e25. https://doi.org/10.1016/j.wombi.2019.05.010

Davis, K., Pearlstein, T., Stuart, S., O'Hara, M. W., & Zlotnick, C. (2013). Analysis of brief screening tools from the detection of postpartum depression: Comparisons of the PRAMS 6-item instrument, PHQ-9, and structured interviews. *Archives of Women's Mental Health, 16*, 271–277.

Declercq, E., Feinberg, E., & Belanoff, C. (2021). Racial inequities in the course of treating perinatal mental health challenges: Results from Listening to Mothers in California. *Birth, 49*, 132–140. https://doi.org/10.1111/birt.12584

Delatte, R., Cao, H., Meltzer-Brody, S., & Menard, M. K. (2009). Universal screening for postpartum depression: An inquiry into provider attitudes and practice. *American Journal of Obstetrics and Gynecology, 200*(5), e63–e64.

Del Castillo, D., & Wright, M. O. (2009). The perils and possibilities in disclosing childhood sexual abuse to a romantic partner. *Journal of Child Sexual Abuse, 18*, 386–404.

Deligiannidis, K. M., & Freeman, M. P. (2014). Complementary and alternative medicine therapies for depression. *Best Practice & Research Clinical Obstetrics & Gynaecology, 28*, 85–95.

Deligiannidis, K. M., Meltzer-Brody, S., Gunduz-Bruce, H., Doherty, J., Jonas, J., Sankoh, A. J., Silber, C., Campbell, A. D., Werneburg, B., Kanes, S. J., & Lasser, R. (2021). Effect of zuranolone vs placebo in postpartum depression: A randomized clinical trial. *JAMA Psychiatry, 78*(9), 951–959. https://doi.org/10.1001/jamapsychiatry.2021.1559

Dell'Aica, I., Caniato, R., Biggin, S., & Garbisa, S. (2007). Matrix proteases, green tea, and St. John's wort: Biomedical research catches up with folk medicine. *Clinica Chimica Acta, 381*, 69–77.

Demissie, Z., Siega-Riz, A. M., Evenson, K. R., Herring, A. H., Dole, N., & Gaynes, B. N. (2011a). Associations between physical activity and postpartum depressive symptoms. *Journal of Women's Health, 20*, 1025–1034.

Demissie, Z., Siega-Riz, A. M., Evenson, K. R., Herring, A. H., Dole, N., & Gaynes, B. N. (2011b). Physical activity and depressive symptoms among pregnant women: The PINS study. *Archives of Women's Mental Health, 14*, 145–157.

Dennis, C.-L. (2004a). Can we identify mothers at risk for postpartum depression in the immediate postpartum period using the Edinburgh Postnatal Depression Scale? *Journal of Affective Disorders, 78*, 163–169.

Dennis, C.-L. (2004b). Influence of depressive symptomatology on maternal health service utilization and general health. *Archives of Women's Mental Health, 7*, 183–191.

Dennis, C.-L., & Allen, K. (2008). Interventions (other than pharmacological, psychosocial or psychological) for treating antenatal depression. *Cochrane Database Systematic Review*, (4), CD006795. https://doi.org/10.001002/14651858.CD14006795.pub14651852.

Dennis, C.-L., & Chung-Lee, L. (2006). Postpartum depression help-seeking barriers and maternal treatment preferences: A qualitative systematic review. *Birth, 33*(4), 323–331.

Dennis, C.-L., Hodnett, E., Kenton, L., Weston, J., Zupancic, J., Stewart, D. E., & Kiss, A. (2009). Effect of peer support on prevention of postnatal depression among high-risk women: Multisite randomised controlled trial. *British Medical Journal, 338*, a3064 https://doi.org/:3010.1136/bmj.a3064

Dennis, C.-L., & Kingston, D. (2008). *Journal of Obstetric, Gynecologic and Neonatal Nursing, 37*, 301–314.

Dennis, C.-L., Merry, L., Stewart, D., & Gagnon, A. J. (2016). Prevalence, continuation, and identification of postpartum depressive symptomatology among refugee, asylum-seeking, non-refugee immigrant, and Canadian-born women: Results from a prospective cohort study. *Archive of Women's Mental Health, 19*, 959–967. https://doi.org/10.1007/s00737-016-0633-5

Desan, P. H., Weinstein, A. J., Michalak, E. E., Tam, E. M., Meesters, Y., Ruiter, M. J., Horn, E., Telner, J., Iskandar, H., Boivin, D. B., & Lam, R. W. (2007). A controlled trial of the Litebook light-emitting diode (LED) light therapy device for treatment of Seasonal Affective Disorder (SAD). *BMC Psychiatry, 7*. https://doi.org/10.1186/1471-1244X/1187/1138

Dhiman, P., Pillai, R. R., Wilson, A. B., Premkumar, N., Bharadwaj, B., Ranjan, V. P., & Rajendiran, S. (2021). Cross-sectional association between vitamin B12 status and probable postpartum depression in Indian women. *BMC Pregnancy and Childbirth, 21*, 146. https://doi.org/10.1186/s12884-021-03622x

Di Pietro, L., Evenson, K. R., Bloodgood, B., Sprow, K., Troiano, R. P., & Piercy, K. L. (2019). Benefits of physical activity during pregnancy and postpartum: An umbrella review. *Medicine & Science in Sports & Exercise, 51*(6), 1292–1302. https://doi.org/10.1249/MSS.0000000000001941

di Scalea, T. L., Hanusa, B. H., & Wisner, K. L. (2009). Sexual function in postpartum women treated for depression: Results from a randomized trial of nortriptyline versus sertraline. *Journal of Clinical Psychiatry, 70*(3), 423–428.

Doering, L. V., Cross, R., Vredevoe, D., Martinez-Maza, O. L., & Cowan, M. J. (2007). Infection, depression and immunity in women after coronary artery bypass: A pilot study of cognitive-behavioral therapy. *Alternative Therapy, Health & Medicine, 13*, 18–21.

Donmez, M., Yorguner, N., Kora, K., & Topcuoglu, V. (2022). Efficacy of bright light therapy in perinatal depression: A randomized, double-blind, placebo-controlled study. *Journal of Psychiatric Research, 149*, 315–322. https://doi.org/10.1016/j.jpsychires.2022.02.027

Downs, D. S., DiNallo, J. M., & Kirner, T. L. (2008). Determinants of pregnancy and postpartum depression: Prospective influences of depressive symptoms, body image satisfaction, and exercise behavior. *Annals of Behavioral Medicine, 36*(1), 54–63.

Dugoua, J.-J., Mills, E., Perri, D., & Koren, G. (2006). Safety and efficacy of St. John's wort (Hypericum) during pregnancy and lactation. *Canadian Journal of Clinical Pharmacology, 13*, e268–e276.

Dunn, C., Hanieh, E., Roberts, R. E., & Powrie, R. (2012). Mindful pregnancy and childbirth: Effects of a mindfulness-based intervention on women's psychological distress and well-being in the perinatal period. *Archives of Women's Mental Health, 15*, 139–143.

Dunstan, J. A., Mori, T. A., Barden, A., Beilin, L. J., Holt, P. G., Calder, P. C., Taylor, A. L., & Prescott, S. L. (2004). Effects of n-3 polyunsaturated fatty acid supplementation in pregnancy on maternal and fetal erythrocyte fatty acid composition. *European Journal of Clinical Nutrition, 58*, 429–437.

Dunstan, J. A., Roper, J., Mitoulas, L., Hartmann, P. E., Simmer, K., & Prescott, S. L. (2004). The effect of supplementation with fish oil during pregnancy on breast milk immunoglobulin A, soluble CD14, cytokine levels and fatty acid composition. *Clinical & Experimental Allergy, 34*, 1237–1242.

Earls, M. F., & The Committee on Psychosocial Aspects of Child and Family Health. (2010). Clinical report incorporating recognition and management of perinatal and postpartum depression into pediatric practice. *Pediatrics.* https://doi.org/10.1542/peds.2010-2348

Eckenrode, J., Campa, M., Luckey, D. W., Henderson, C. R., Cole, R., Kitzman, H., Anson, E., Sidora-Arcoleo, K., Powers, J., & Olds, D. (2010). Long-term effects of prenatal and infancy nurse home visitation on the life course of youths. *Archives of Pediatric & Adolescent Medicine, 164*(1), 9–15.

Edwards, R. C., Thullen, M. J., Korfmacher, J., Lantos, J. D., Henson, L. G., & Hans, S. L. (2013). Breastfeeeding and complementary food: Randomized trial of community doula home visiting. *Pediatrics, 132*(S2), S160–166. https://doi.org/10.1542/peds.2013-1021P

Einarson, A., Choi, J., Einarson, T. R., & Koren, G. (2009). Rates of spontaneous and therapeutic abortions following use of antidepressants in pregnancy: Results from a large prospective database. *Journal of Obstetrics and Gynaecology Canada, 31*(5), 452–456.

El Marroun, H., Jaddoe, V. V. W., Hudziak, J. J., Roza, S. J., Steegers, E. A. P., Hofman, A., Verhulst, F. C., White, T. J. H., Stricker, B. H. C., & Tiemeier, H. (2012). Maternal use of selective-serotonin reuptake inhibitors, fetal growth, and risk of adverse birth outcomes. *Archives of General Psychiatry, 69*, 706–714.

Emery, C. F., Kiecolt-Glaser, J. K., Glaser, R., Malarky, W. B., & Frid, D. J. (2005). Exercise accelerates wound healing among health older adults: A preliminary investigation. *The Journals of Gerontology: Medical Sciences, 60A*, 1432–1436.

Erman, M. K. (2007). Pharamcologic therapy: Melatonin, antidepressants, and other agents. *Primary Psychiatry, 14*, 21–24.

Ernst, E. (2002). The risk-benefit profile of commonly used herbal therapies: Ginkgo, St. John's wort, ginseng, echinacea, saw palmetto, and kava. *Annals of Internal Medicine, 136*, 42–53.

Ertan, D., Hingray, C., Burlacu, E., Sterle, A., & El-Hage, W. (2021). Posttraumatic stress disorder following childbirth. *BMC Psychiatry, 21*. https://doi.org/10.1186/s12888-021-03158-6

Eustis, E. H., Ernst, S., Sutton, K., & Battle, C. L. (2019). Innovations in the treatment of perinatal depression: The role of yoga and physical activity interventions during pregnancy and postpartum. *Current Psychiatry Reports, 21*(12), 133. https://doi.org/10.1007/s11920-019-1121-1

Evans, M., Donelle, L., & Hume-Loveland, L. (2012). Social support and online postpartum discussion groups: A content analysis. *Patient Education and Counseling, 87*, 405–410.

Fantasia, H. C. (2019). Brexanolone is the first drug specifically for postpartum depression. *Nursing for Women's Health, 23*(5). https://doi.org/10.1016/jmnwh.2019.07.004

Fellmeth, G., Plugge, E., Fazel, M., Nosten, S., Oo, M. M., Pimanpanarak, M., Phichitpadungtham, Y., Fitzpatrick, R., & McGready, R. (2021). Perinatal depression in migrant and refugee women on the Thai-Myanmar border: Does social support matter? *Philosophical Transactions of the Royal Society, 376*. https://doi.org/10.1098/rstb.2020.0030

Fernandez y Garcia, E., Joseph, J., Wilson, M. D., Hinton, L., Simon, G., Ludman, E. J., Scott, F., & Kravitz, R. L. (2015). Pediatric-based intervention to motivate mothers to seek follow-up for depression screens: The Motivating Our Mothers (MOM) trial. *Academic Pediatrics, 15*, 311–318.

Ferrucci, L., Cherubini, A., Bandinelli, S., Bartali, B., Corsi, A., Lauretani, F., Martin, A., Andres-Lacueva, C., Senin, U., & Guralnik, J. M. (2006). Relationship of plasma polyunsaturated fatty acids to circulating inflammatory markers. *Journal of Clinical Endocrinology & Metabolism, 91*, 439–446.

Filardi, T., Vari, R., Ferretti, E., Zicari, A., Morano, S., & Santangelo, C. (2020). Curcumin: Could this compound be useful in pregnancy and pregnancy-related complications? *Nutrients, 12*(10). https://doi.org/10.3390/nu12103179

First, M. B., & Gibbon, M. (2004). The structured clinical interview for DSM-IV axis I disorders (SCID-I) and the structured clinical interviews: A meta-research review. *BMC Medicine, 17*(1). https://doi.org/10.1186/s12916-019-1297-6

Fisher, S. D., Kopelman, R., & O'Hara, M. W. (2012). Partner report of paternal depression using the Edinburgh Postnatal Depression Scale-Partner. *Archives of Women's Mental Health, 15,* 283–288.

Foa, E. B., & Cahill, S. P. (2002). Specialized treatment for PTSD: Matching survivors to the appropriate modality. In R. Yehuda (Ed.), *Treating trauma survivors with PTSD* (pp. 43–62). American Psychiatric Association Press.

Forsyth, J., Boath, E., Henshaw, C., & Brown, H. (2017). Exercise as an adjunct treatment for postpartum depression for women living in an inner city: A pilot study. *Health Care for Women International, 38*(6), 635–639. https://doi.org/10.1080/07399332.2017.1295049

Frangou, S., Lewis, M., & McCrone, P. (2006). Efficacy of ethyl-eicosapentaenoic acid in bipolar depression: Randomized double-blind placebo-controlled study. *British Journal of Psychiatry, 188,* 46–50.

Freeman, M. P. (2007). Antenatal depression: Navigating the treatment dilemmas. *American Journal of Psychiatry, 164,* 1162–1165.

Freeman, M. P., Fava, M., Lake, J., Trivedi, M. H., Wisner, K. L., & Mischoulon, D. (2010). Complementary and alternative medicine in major depressive disorder: The American Psychiatric Association Task Force Report. *Journal of Clinical Psychiatry, 71*(6), 669–681.

Freeman, M. P., Hibbeln, J. R., Wisner, K. L., Brumbach, B. H., Watchman, M., & Gelenberg, A. J. (2006b). Randomized dose-ranging pilot trial of omega-3 fatty acids for postpartum depression. *Acta Psychiatrica Scandanavica, 113,* 31–35.

Freeman, M. P., Hibbeln, J. R., Wisner, K. L., Davis, J. M., Mischoulon, D., Peet, M., Keck, P. E. J., Marangell, L. B., Richardson, A. J., Lake, J., & Stoll, A. L. (2006a). Omega-3 fatty acids: Evidence basis for treatment and future research in psychiatry. *Journal of Clinical Psychiatry, 67,* 1954–1967.

Freeman, M. P., Wright, R., Watchman, M., Wahl, R. A., Sisk, D. J., Fraleigh, L., & Weibrecht, J. M. (2005). Postpartum depression assessments at well-baby visits: Screening feasibility, prevalence, and risk factors. *Journal of Women's Health, 14*(10), 929–935.

Fregni, F., El-Hagrassy, M. M., Pacheco-Barrios, K., Carvalho, S., Leite, J., & Simis, M. (2021). Evidence-based guidelines and secondary meta-analysis for the use of transcranial direct current stimulation in neurological and psychiatric disorders. *International Journal of Neuropsychopharmacology, 24*(4), 256–313. https://doi.org/10.1093/ijnp/pyaa051

Frey, B. N., Simpson, W., Wright, L., & Steiner, M. (2012). Sensitivity and specificity of the Mood Disorder Questionnaire as a screening tool for bipolar disorder during pregnancy and the postpartum period. *Journal of Clinical Psychiatry, 73*(11), 1456–1461. https://doi.org/10.4088/JCP.12m07856

Friedman, M. J. (2001). *Posttraumatic stress disorder: The latest assessment and treatment strategies.* Compact Clinicals.

Friedman, M. J., Cohen, J. A., Foa, E. B., & Keane, T. M. (2009). Integration and summary. In E. B. Foa, T. M. Keane, M. J. Friedman, & J. A. Cohen (Eds.), *Effective treatments for PTSD: Practice guidelines from the International Society for Traumatic Stress Studies* (pp. 617–642). Guilford.

Fuemmeler, B. F., Yang, C., Costanzo, P., Hoyle, R. H., Siegler, I. C., Williams, R. B., & Ostbye, T. (2012). Parenting styles and body mass index trajectories from adolescence to adulthood. *Health Psychology, 31*(4), 441–449.

Fusar-Poli, L., Vozza, L., Gabbiadini, A., Vanella, A., Concas, I., Tinacci, S., Petralia, A., Signorelli, M. S., & Aguglia, E. (2020). Curcumin for depression: A meta-analysis. *Critical Reviews in Food Science and Nutrition, 60*(15), 2643–2653. https://doi.org/10.1080/10408398.2019.1653260

Gagnon, A. J., & Stewart, D. E. (2014). Resilience in international migrant women following violence associated with pregnancy. *Archives of Women's Mental Health*, 17, 303–310. https://doi.org/10.1007/s00737-013-0392-5

Gamble, J. A., Creedy, D., Webster, J., & Moyle, W. (2002). A review of the literature on debriefing or non-directive counseling to prevent postpartum emotional distress. *Midwifery*, 8(1), 72–79.

Garbazza, C., Cirgnotta, F., D'Agostino, A., Cicolin, A., Hackethal, S., Wirz-Justice, A., Cajochen, C., Manconi, M., & "Life-ON" Study Group. (2022). Sustained remission from perinatal depression after bright light therapy: A pilot randomised, placebo-controlled trial. *Acta Psychiatrica Scandinavia*, 146(4), 350–356. https://doi.org/10.1111/acps.13482

Gehlen, M., Lazarescu, A. D., Hinz, C., Schwarz-Eywill, M., Pfeifer, M., Balasingam, S., & Maier, A. (2019). Long-term outcome of patients with pregnancy and lactation-associated osteoporosis (PLO) with a particular focus on quality of life. *Clinical Rheumatology*, 38(12), 3575–3583. https://doi.org/10.1007/s10067-019-04758-0

Gerbasi, M. E., Meltzer-Brody, S., Acaster, S., Fridman, M., Bonthapally, V., Hodkins, P., Kanes, S. J., & Eldar-Lissai, A. (2021). Brexanolone in postpartum depression: Post hoc analyses to help inform clinical decision making. *Journal of Women's Health*, 20(3), 385–392. https://doi.org/10.1089/jwh.2020.8483

Gildner, T. E., Uwizeye, G., Milner, R. L., Alston, G. C., & Thayer, Z. M. (2021). Associations between postpartum depression and assistance with household tasks and childcare during the COVID-19 pandemic: Evidence from American mothers. *BMC Pregnancy and Childbirth*, 21. https://doi.org/10.1186/s12884-021-04300-8

Gjerdingen, D., Crow, S., McGovern, P., Miner, M., & Center, B. (2009). Postpartum depression screening at well-child visits: Validity of a 2-question screen and the PHQ-9. *Annals of Family Medicine*, 7(1), 63–70.

Glover, V., Onozawa, K., & Hodgkinson, A. (2002). Benefits of infant massage for mothers with postnatal depression. *Seminars in Neonatology*, 7, 495–500.

Golden, R. N., Gaynes, B. N., Ekstrom, R. D., Hamer, R. M., Jacobsen, F. M., Suppes, T., Wisner, K. L., & Nemeroff, C. B. (2005). The efficacy of light therapy in the treatment of mood disorders: A review and meta-analysis of the evidence. *American Journal of Psychiatry*, 162, 656–662.

Goodman, J. H., Guarino, A., Chenausky, K., Klein, L., Prager, J., Petersen, K. L., Forget, A., & Freeman, M. (2014). CALM pregnancy: Results of a pilot study of mindfulness-based cognitive therapy for perinatal anxiety. *Archives of Women's Mental Health*, 17, 373–387.

Goyal, M., Singh, S., Sibinga, E. M. S., Gould, N. F., Rowland-Seymour, A., Sharma, R., & Berger, Z. (2014). *Meditation programs for psychological stress and well-being* (Vol. 13(14)-EHC116-EF). Agency for Healthcare Research and Quality.

Grandjean, P., Bjerve, K. S., Weihe, P., & Steuerwald, U. (2001). Birthweight in a fishing community: Significance of essential fatty acids and marine food contaminants. *International Journal of Epidemiology*, 30, 1272–1278.

Griffin, L. D., & Mellon, S. H. (1999). Selective-serotonin reuptake inhibitors directly alter activity of neurosteroidogenic enzymes. *Proceedings of the National Academy of Science*, 96(23), 13512–13517. https://doi.org/10.1073/pnas.96.23.13512

Grigoriadis, S., Graves, L., Peer, M., Mamisashvili, L., Tomlinson, G., Vigod, S. N., Dennis, C.-L., Steiner, M., Brown, C., Cheung, A., Dawson, H., Rector, N. A., Guenette, M., & Richter, M. (2018). Maternal anxiety during pregnancy and the association with adverse perinatal outcomes: Systematic review and meta-analysis. *Journal of Clinical Psychiatry*, 79(5), 17r12011. https://doi.org/10.4088/JCP.17r12011

Grigoriadis, S., & Ravitz, P. (2007). An approach to interpersonal psychotherapy for postpartum depression: Focusing on interpersonal changes. *Canadian Family Physician*, 53, 1469–1475.

Grzeskowiak, L. E., Morrison, J. L., Henriksen, T. B., Bech, B. H., Obel, C., Olsen, J., & Pedersen, L. H. (2015). Prenatal antidepressant exposure and child behavioural outcomes at 7 years of age: A study within the Danish National Birth Cohort. *British Journal of Obstetrics & Gynaecology*, 123(12). https://doi.org/10.1111/1471-0528.13611

Guo, L., Zhang, J., Mu, L., & Ye, Z. (2020). Preventing postpartum depression with mindful self-compassion intervention. *Journal of Nervous & Mental Disease, 208*, 100–107. https://doi.org/10.1097/NMD.0000000000001096

Hagaman, A., LeMasters, K., Zivich, P. N., Sikander, S., Bates, L. M., Bhalotra, S., Chung, E., Zaidi, A., & Maselko, J. (2021). Longitudinal effects of perinatal social support on maternal depression: A marginal structural modelling approach. *Journal of Epidemiology & Community Health, 75*(10), 936–943. https://doi.org/10.1136/jech-2020-215836

Hagan, R., Evans, S. F., & Pope, S. (2004). Preventing postnatal depression in mothers of very preterm infants: A randomized controlled trial. *British Journal of Obstetrics & Gynecology, 111*, 641–647.

Hale, T. W. (2021). *Hales's medications and mothers' milk* (19th ed.). Springer Publishing.

Hale, T. W., Kendall-Tackett, K. A., Cong, Z., Votta, R., & McCurdy, F. (2010). Discontinuation syndrome in newborns whose mothers took antidepressants while pregnant or breastfeeding. *Breastfeeding Medicine, 5*, 283–288.

Hallahan, B., & Garland, M. R. (2005). Essential fatty acids and mental health. *British Journal of Psychiatry, 186*, 275–277.

Hallahan, B., Hibbeln, J. R., Davis, J. M., & Garland, M. R. (2007). Omega-3 fatty acid supplementation in patients with recurrent self-harm. Single-centre double-blind randomized controlled trial. *British Journal of Psychiatry, 190*, 118–122.

Haller, H., Anheyer, D., Cramer, H., & Dobos, G. (2019). Complementary therapies for clinical depression: An overview of systematic reviews. *BMJ Open, 9*(8). https://doi.org/10.1136/bmjopen-2018-028527

Hamazaki, K., Itomura, M., Huan, M., Nishizawa, H., Sawazaki, S., Tanouchi, M., Watanabe, S., Hamazaki, T., Terasawa, K., & Yazawa, K. (2005). Effect of omega-3 fatty acid-containing phospholipids on blood catecholamine concentrations in healthy volunteers: A randomized, placebo-controlled, double-blind trial. *Nutrition, 21*, 705–710.

Hamer, M., & Steptoe, A. (2007). Association between physical fitness, parasympathetic control, and proinflammatory responses to mental stress. *Psychosomatic Medicine, 69*, 660–666.

Handal, M., Skurtveit, S., Furu, K., Hernandez-Diaz, S., Skovlund, E., Nystad, W., & Selmer, R. (2016). Motor development in children prenatally exposed to selective-serotonin reuptake inhibitors: A large population-based pregnancy cohort study. *British Journal of Obstetrics & Gynaecology, 123*(12), 1908–1917. https://doi.org/10.1111/1471-0528.13582

Hanusa, B. H., Scholle, S. H., Haskett, R. F., Spadaro, K., & Wisner, K. L. (2008). Screening for depression in the postpartum period: A comparison of three instruments. *Journal of Women's Health (Larchmont), 17*(4), 585–596. https://doi.org/10.1089/jwh.2006.0248

Harkness, R., & Bratman, S. (2003). *Handbook of drug-herb and drug-supplement interactions.* Mosby.

Head, J. G., Storfer-Isser, A., O'Connor, K. G., Hoagwood, K. E., Kelleher, K. J., Heneghan, A. M., Park, E. R., Chaudron, L. H., Stein, M. B., & Horwitz, S. M. (2008). Does education influence pediatricians' perceptions of physician-specific barriers for maternal depression? *Clinical Pediatrics, 47*, 670–678.

Heck, J. L. (2018). Screening for postpartum depression in American Indian/Alaska Native women: A comparison of instruments. *American Indian and Alaska Native Mental Health Research, 25*, 74–102. https://doi.org/10.5820/aian.2502.2018.74

Heh, S. S., Huang, L. H., Ho, S. M., Fu, Y. Y., & Wang, L. L. (2008). Effectiveness of an exercise support program in reducing the severity of postnatal depression in Taiwanese women. *Birth, 35*(1), 60–65.

Heinrichs, M., Meinlschmidt, G., Neumann, I., Wagner, S., Kirschbaum, C., Ehlert, U., & Hellhammer, D. H. (2001). Effects of suckling on hypothalamic-pituitary-adrenal axis responses to psychosocial stress in postpartum lactating women. *Journal of Clinical Endocrinology & Metabolism, 86*, 4798–4804.

Heise, A. M., & Wiessinger, D. (2011). Dysphoric milk ejection reflex: A case report. *International Breastfeeding Journal*, 6(6).

Helland, I. B., Smith, L., Saarem, K., Saugstad, O. D., & Drevon, C. A. (2003). Maternal supplementation with very-long-chain n-3 fatty acids during pregnancy and lactation augments children's IQ at 4 years of age. *Pediatrics*, 111, e39–e44.

Heneghan, A. M., Chaudron, L. H., Storfer-Isser, A., Park, E. R., Kelleher, K. J., Stein, R. E. K., Hoagwood, K. E., O'Connor, K. G., & McCue Horwitz, S. (2007). Factors associated with identification and management or maternal depression by pediatricians. *Pediatrics*, 119, 44–454.

Hibbeln, J. R. (2002). Seafood consumption, the DHA content of mothers' milk and prevalence rates of postpartum depression: A cross-national, ecological analysis. *Journal of Affective Disorders*, 69, 15–29.

Hilt, R. J. (2015). Postpartum depression screening. *Pediatric Annals*, 44, 346–347.

Hirschfeld, R. M., Williams, J. B., Spitzer, R. L., Calabrese, J. R., Flynn, L., Keck, P. E. J., McElroy, S. L., Post, R. M., Rapport, D. J., Russell, J. M., Sachs, G. S., & Zajecka, J. (2000). Development and validation of a screening instrument for bipolar spectrum disorder: The Mood Disorder Questionnaire. *American Journal of Psychiatry*, 157(111), 1873–1875. https://doi.org/10.1176/appi.ajp.157.11.1873

Howell, L. M., Bodnar-Deren, S., Balbierz, A., London, H., Mora, P. A., Zlotnick, C., Wang, J., & Leventhal, H. (2014). An intervention to reduce postpartum depressive symptoms: A randomized controlled trial. *Archives of Women's Mental Health*, 17, 57–63.

Hu, Z. P., Yang, X. X., Chan, S. Y., Xu, A. L., Duan, W., Zhu, Y. Z., Sheu, F.-S., Boelsterli, U. A., Chan, E., Zhang, Q., Wang, J.-C., Rachel Ee, P. L., Koh, H. L., Huang, M., & Zhou, S.-F. (2006). St. John's wort attenuates irinotecan-induced diarrhea via down-regulation of intestinal pro-inflammatory cytokines and inhibition of intestinal epithelial apoptosis. *Toxicology & Applied Pharmacology*, 216, 225–237.

Huang, X., Zhuo, Y., Wang, X., Xu, J., Yang, Z., Zhou, Y., Lv, H., Ma, X., Yan, B., Zhao, H., & Yu, H. (2023). Structural and functional improvement of amygdala subregions in postpartum depression after acupuncture. *Frontiers in Human Neuroscience*, 17. https://doi.org/10.3389/fnhum.2023.1163746

Humphrey, S. (2007). Herbal therapeutics during lactation. In T. W. Hale & P. E. Hartmann (Eds.), *Textbook of human lactation* (pp. 629–654). Hale Publishing.

Hung, K. J., Tomilson, M., Le Roux, I. M., Dewing, S., Chopra, M., & Tsai, A. C. (2014). Community-based prenatal screening for postpartum depression in a South African township. *International Journal of Gynaecology and Obstetrics*, 126(1), 74–77. https://doi.org/10.1016/j.ijgo.2014.01.011

Hypericum Depression Trial Study Group. (2002). Effect of Hypericum perforatum (St. John's Wort) in major depressive disorder. *Journal of the American Medical Association*, 287, 1807–1814.

Irwin, M. R., Olmstead, R., Carrillo, C., Sadeghi, N., Breen, E. C., Witarama, T., & Yokomizo, M. (2014). Cognitive-behavioral therapy vs. Tai Chi for late life insomnia and inflammatory risk: A randomized controlled comparative efficacy trial. *Sleep*, 37, 1543–1552.

Jia-Hui, M., Sai-Ying, W., He-Ya, Y., Dan-Yang, L., Shi-Chao, L., Shan-Shan, Z., Li-Fei, W., & Kai-Ming, D. (2019). Prophylactic use of ketamine reduces postpartum depression in Chinese women undergoing cesarean section. *Psychiatry Research*, 279, 252–258. https://doi.org/10.1016/j.psychres.2019.03.026

Kabir, K., Sheeder, J., & Kelly, L. S. (2008). Identifying postpartum depression: Are 3 questions as good as 10? *Pediatrics*, 122, e696–e702.

Kallen, B. (2004). Neonate characteristics after maternal use of antidepressants in late pregnancy. *Archives of Pediatric & Adolescent Medicine*, 158, 312–316.

Kantamneni, S. (2015). Cross-talk and regulation between glutamate and GABA-B receptors. *Frontiers in Cellular Neuroscience*, 9. http://doi.org/10.3389/fncel.2015.00135.

Kearney, D. J., McDermott, K., Malte, C., Martinez, M., & Simpson, T. L. (2013). Effects of participation in a mindfulness program for veterans with posttraumatic stress disorder: A randomized controlled pilot study. *Journal of Clinical Psychology, 69,* 14–27.

Kelmendi, B., Adams, T. G., Southwick, S. M., Abdallah, C. G., & Krystal, J. H. (2017). Posttraumatic stress disorder: An integrated overview of the neurobiological rationale for pharmacology. *Clinical Psychology: Science and Practice, 24*(3), 281–297. https://doi.org/10.1111/cpsp.12202

Kendall-Tackett, K. A. (2007). A new paradigm for depression in new mothers: The central role of inflammation and how breastfeeding and anti-inflammatory treatments protect maternal mental health. *International Breastfeeding Journal, 2,* 6. https://doi.org/10.1186/1746-4358-2-6

Kendall-Tackett, K. A. (2017). *Depression in new mothers* (3rd ed.). Routledge.

Kendall-Tackett, K. A., & Hale, T. W. (2010). The use of antidepressants in pregnant and breastfeeding women: A review of recent studies. *Journal of Human Lactation, 26*(2), 187–196.

Kiecolt-Glaser, J. K., Belury, M. A., Porter, K., Beversdoft, D., Lemeshow, S., & Glaser, R. (2007). Depressive symptoms, omega-6: omega-3 fatty acids, and inflammation in older adults. *Psychosomatic Medicine, 69,* 217–224.

Kiecolt-Glaser, J. K., Christian, L., Preston, H., Houts, C., Malarkey, W. B., Emery, C. F., & Glaser, R. (2010). Stress, inflammation, and yoga practice. *Psychosomatic Medicine, 72*(2), 113–121.

Kiecolt-Glaser, J. K., Derry, H. M., & Fagundes, C. P. (2015). Inflammation: Depression fans the flames and feasts on the heat. *American Journal of Psychiatry, 172*(11), 1075–1091. https://doi.org/10.1176/appi.ajp.2015.15020152

Kiecolt-Glaser, J. K., Loving, T. J., Stowell, J. R., Malarky, W. B., Lemeshow, S., Dickinson, S. L., & Glaser, R. (2005). Hostile marital interactions, proinflammatory cytokine production, and wound healing. *Archives of General Psychiatry, 62,* 1377–1384.

Kim, J. J., LaPorte, L. M., Adams, M. G., Gordon, T. E. J., Kuendig, J. M., & Silver, R. K. (2009). Obstetric care provider engagement in a perinatal depression screening program. *Archives of Women's Mental Health, 12,* 167–172.

Kim, S. H., Schneider, S. M., Kravitz, L., Mermier, C., & Burge, M. R. (2013). Mind-body practices for posttraumatic stress disorder. *Journal of Investigative Medicine, 61,* 827–834.

Kim, Y.-D., Heo, I., Shin, B.-C., Crawford, C., Kang, H.-W., & Lim, J.-H. (2013). Acupuncture for posttraumatic stress disorder: A systematic review of randomized controlled trials and prospective clinical trials. *Evidence-Based Complementary and Alternative Medicine.* http://dx.doi.org/10.1155/2013/615857

Kimmel, M. C., Cox, E. Q., Schiller, C., Gettes, E., & Meltzer-Brody, S. (2018). Pharmacologic treatment of perinatal depression. *Obstetrics & Gynecology Clinics, 45*(1), 419-440.

King, P. A. (2012). Replicability of structural models of the Edinburgh Postnatal Depression Scale (EPDS) in a community sample of postpartum African American women with low socioeconomic status. *Archives of Women's Mental Health, 15,* 77–86.

Klier, C. M., Schafer, M. R., Schmid-Siegel, B., Lenz, G., & Mannel, M. (2002). St. John's wort (Hypericum Perforatum) – Is it safe during breastfeeding? *Pharmacopsychiatry, 35,* 29–30.

Klier, C. M., Schmid-Siegel, B., Schafer, M. R., Lenz, G., Saria, A., Lee, A., & Zernig, G. (2006). St. John's wort (Hypericum perforatum) and breastfeeding: Plasma and breast milk concentrations of hyperforin for 5 mothers and 2 infants. *Journal of Clinical Psychiatry, 67,* 305–309.

Ko, Y.-L., Yang, C.-L., Fang, C.-L., Lee, M.-Y., & Lin, P.-C. (2013). Community-based postpartum exercise program. *Journal of Clinical Nursing, 22,* 2122–2131.

Kobayashi, K., Tsugami, Y., Suzuki, N., Suzuki, T., & Nishimura, T. (2021). Suppressive effects of curcumin on milk production without inflammatory responses in lactating mammary epithelial cells. *Phytomedicine, 80.* https://doi.org/10.1016/j.phymed.2020.153360

Kobayashi, M., Ogawa, K., Morisaki, N., Tani, Y., Horikawa, R., & Fujiwara, T. (2017). Dietary n-3 polyunsaturated fatty acids in late pregnancy and postpartum depressive symptoms among Japanese women. *Frontiers in Psychiatry, 8.* https://doi.org/10.3389/fpsyt.2017.00241

Kocak, V., Ege, E., & Iyisoy, M. S. (2021). The development of the postpartum mobile support application and the effect of the application on mothers' anxiety and depression symptoms. *Archives of Psychiatric Nursing, 35*, 441–449. https://doi.org/10.1016/j.apnu.2021.06.009

Koopman, C., Ismailji, T., Holmes, D., Classen, C. C., Palesh, O., & Wales, T. (2005). The effects of expressive writing on pain, depression and posttraumatic stress disorder symptoms in survivors of intimate partner violence. *Journal of Health Psychology, 10*(2), 211–221.

Kristensen, J. H., Ilett, K. F., Rampono, J., Kohan, R., & Hackett, L. P. (2006). Transfer of the antidepressant mirtazapine into breast milk. *British Journal of Clinical Pharmacology, 63*(3), 322–327.

Kroenke, K., Spitzer, R. L., & Williams, J. B. (2001). The PHQ-9: Validity of a brief depression severity measure. *Journal of General Internal Medicine, 16*, 606–613.

Kroenke, K., Spitzer, R. L., Williams, J. B. W., & Lowe, B. (2009). An ultra-brief screening scale for anxiety and depression: The PHQ-4. *Psychosomatics, 50*, 613–621.

Kronenfeld, N., Berlin, M., Shaniv, D., & Berkovitch, M. (2017). Use of psychotropic medications in breastfeeding women. *Birth Defects Research, 109*, 967–997. https://doi.org/10.1002/bdr2.1077

Kroska, E. B., & Stowe, Z. (2020). Postpartum depression: Identification and treatment in the clinic setting. *Obstetric & Gynecology Clinics of North America, 47*, 409–419. https://doi.org/10.1016/j.ogc.2020.05.001

Kryst, J., Kawalec, P., & Pilc, A. (2020). Efficacy and safety of intranasal esketamine for the treatment of major depressive disorder. *Expert Opinions in Pharmacotherapy, 21*(1), 9–20. https://doi.org/10.1080/14656566.2019.1683161

Kuhn, M. A., & Winston, D. (2000). *Herbal therapy and supplements: A scientific and traditional approach*. Lippincott.

LactMed. (2021). Drugs and lactation database. *St. John's wort*. www.ncbi.nlm.nih.gov/books/NBK501922

Lam, R. W., Song, C., & Yatham, L. N. (2004). Does neuroimmune dysfunction mediate seasonal mood changes in winter depression? *Medical Hypotheses, 63*, 567–573.

Lane, A. M., Crone-Grant, D., & Lane, H. (2002). Mood changes following exercise. *Perceptual & Motor Skills, 94*, 732–734.

Lang, E., Colquhoun, H., LeBlanc, J. C., Riva, J. J., Moore, A., Traversy, G., Wilson, B., Grad, R., & Canadian Task Force on Preventive Health Care. (2022). Recommendation on instrument-based screening for depression during pregnancy and the postpartum period. *Canadian Medical Association Journal, 194*(28), E981–E989. https://doi.org/10.1503/cmaj.220290

Lappin, J. (2001). Time points for assessing perinatal mood must be optimized. *British Medical Journal, 323*, 1367a.

Larsen, A., Pintye, J., Obhiambo, B., Mwongeli, N., Marwa, M. M., Watoyi, S., Kinuthia, J., Abuna, F., Gomez, L., Dettinger, J., Bhat, A., & John-Stewart, G. J. (2023). Comparing depression screening tools (CESD-10, EPDS, PHQ-9, and PHQ-2) for diagnostic performance and epidemiologic association is among postpartum Kenyan women: Implications for research and practice. *Journal of Affective Disorders, 324*, 637–644. https://doi.org/10.1016/j.jad.2022.12.101

Laurin, A., Nard, N., Dalmont, M., Sulteau, S., Benard, C., & Bonnot, O. (2022). Efficacy and safety of transcranial electric stimulation during the perinatal period: A systematic literature review and three case reports. *Journal of Clinical Medicine, 11*(14), 4048. https://doi.org/10.3390/jcm11144048

Lawvere, S., & Mahoney, M. C. (2005). St. John's wort. *American Family Physician, 72*, 2249–2254.

Leboffe, E. N., Pietragallo, H. C., Liu, G., Ba, D., Leslie, D., & Chuang, C. H. (2023). The impact of the 2015 ACOG screening guidelines on the diagnosis of postpartum depression among privately insured women. *328*, 103–107. https://doi.org/10.1016/j.jad.2023.02.020

LeCheminant, J. D., Hinman, T., Pratt, K. B., Earl, N., Bailey, B. W., Thackerary, R., & Tucker, L. A. (2014). Effect of resistance training on body composition, self-efficacy, depression, and activity in postpartum women. *Scandinavian Journal of Medical Science of Sports, 159*, 1361–1366.

Lecrubier, Y., Clerc, G., Didi, R., & Kieser, M. (2002). Efficacy of St. John's wort extract WS 5570 in major depression: A double-blind, placebo-controlled trial. *American Journal of Psychiatry*, *159*, 1361–1366.

Lee, C., Crawford, C., Wallerstedt, D., York, A., Duncan, A., Smith, J., Sprengel, M., Welton, R., & Jonas, W. (2012). The effectiveness of acupuncture research across components of the trauma spectrum response (TSR): A systematic review of reviews. *Systematic Reviews*, *1*, 49. www.systematicreviewsjournal.com/content/1/1/46

Lefaucheur, J.-P., Aleman, A., Baeken, C., Benninger, D. H., Brunelin, J., & Di Lazzaro, V. (2020). Evidence-based guidelines on the therapeutic use of repetitive transcranial magnetic stimulation (rTMS): An update (2014–2018). *Clinical Neurophysiology*, *131*(2), 474–528. https://doi.org/10.1016/j.clinph.2019.11.002

Leger, J., & Letourneau, N. (2015). New mothers and postpartum depression: A narrative review of peer support intervention studies. *Health and Social Care in the Community*, *23*(4), 337–348. https://doi.org/10.1111/hsc.12125

LeMasters, K., Andrabi, N., Zalla, L., Hagaman, A., Chung, E. O., Gallis, J. A., Turner, E. L., Bhalotra, S., Sikander, S., & Maselko, J. (2020). Maternal depression in rural Pakistan: The protective associations with cultural postpartum practices. *BMC Public Health*, *20*(1), 68. https://doi.org/10.1186/s12889-020-8176-0

Leonard, B. E. (2010). The concept of depression as a dysfunction of the immune system. *Current Immunology Review*, *6*(3), 205–212.

Lesperance, F., & Frasure-Smith, N. (2000). Depression in patients with cardiac disease: A practical review. *Journal of Psychosomatic Research*, *48*, 379–391.

Letourneau, N., Duffett-Leger, L., Stewart, M., Hegadoren, K., Dennis, C.-L., Rinaldi, C. M., & Stoppard, J. (2007). Canadian mothers' perceived support needs during postpartum depression. *Journal of Obstetric, Gynecologic, and Neonatal Nursing*, *36*, 441–449.

Leu, S. J., Shiah, I. S., Yatham, L. N., Cheu, Y. M., & Lam, R. W. (2001). Immune-inflammatory markers in patients with seasonal affective disorder: Effects of light therapy. *Journal of Affective Disorders*, *63*, 27–34.

Levis, B., Negeri, Z., Sun, Y., Benedetti, A., & Thombs, B. D. (2020). Accuracy of the Edinburgh Postnatal Depression Scale (EPDS) to detect major depression among pregnant and postpartum women: A systematic review and meta-analysis of individual participant data. *British Medical Journal*, *371*, m4022. https://doi.org/10.1136/bmj.m4022

Li, W., Yin, P., Lao, L., & Xu, S. (2019). Effectiveness of acupuncture used for the management of postpartum depression: A systematic review and meta-analysis. *Biomedical Research International*, *2019*, 6597503. https://doi.org/10.1155/2019/6597503

Li, Y., Zhao, Q., Cross, W. M., Chen, J., Qin, C., & Sun, M. (2020). Assessing the quality of mobile applications targeting postpartum depression in China. *International Journal of Mental Health Nursing*, *29*, 772–785. https://doi.org/10.1111/inm.12713

Lin, P., & Su, K.-P. (2007). A meta-analysis review of double-blinded, placebo-controlled trials of antidepressant efficacy of omega-3 fatty acids. *Journal of Clinical Psychiatry*, *68*(7), 1056–1061.

Lin, P.-Z., Xue, J.-M., Yang, B., Li, M., & Cao, F.-L. (2018). Effectiveness of self-help psychological intervention for treating and preventing postpartum depression. *Archives of Women's Mental Health*, *21*, 491–503. https://doi.org/10.1007/s00737-018-0835-0

Lindensmith, R. (2018). Interventions to improve maternal-infant relationships in mothers with postpartum mood disorders. *MCN American Journal of Maternal-Child Nursing*, *43*(6), 334–340. https://doi.org/10.1097/NMC.0000000000000471

Logsdon, M. C., Wisner, K. L., & Hanusa, B. H. (2009). Does maternal role functioning improve with antidepressant treatment in women with postpartum depression. *Journal of Women's Health*, *18*(1), 85–90.

Looper, K. J. (2007). Potential medical and surgical complications of serotonergic antidepressant medications. *Psychosomatics*, *48*, 1–9.

Lopresti, A. L., Maes, M., Maker, G. L., Hood, S. D., & Drummond, S. (2014). Curcumin for the treatment of major depression: A randomised, double-blind, placebo-controlled study. *Journal of Affective Disorders*, *167*, 368–375. http://dx.doi.org/10.1016/j.jad.2014.06.001

Louik, C., Lin, A. E., Werler, M. M., Hernandez-Diaz, S., & Mitchell, A. A. (2007). First-trimester use of selective-serotonin-reuptake inhibitors and the risk of birth defects. *New England Journal of Medicine*, *356*, 2675–2683.

Lowe, B., Wahl, I., Rose, M., Spitzer, C., Glaesmer, H., Wingenfeld, K., Schneider, A., & Brahler, E. (2010). A 4-item measure of depression and anxiety: Validation and standardization of the Patient Health Questionnaire-4 (PHQ-4) in the general population. *Journal of Affective Disorders*, *122*(1–2), 86–95. https://doi.org/0.1016/j.jad.2009.06.019

Luscher, B., & Mohler, H. (2019). Brexanolone, a neurosteroid antidepressant, vindicates the GABAergic deficit hypothesis of depression and may foster resilience. *F1000Reseach*, *8*, 10.12688/f1000research. 18758.1

Lyubenova, A., Neupane, D., Levis, B., Wu, Y., Sun, Y., He, C., & Thombs, B. D. (2021). Depression prevalence based on the Edinburgh Postnatal Depression Scale compared to Structured Clinical Interview for DSM Disorders classification: Systematic review and individual participant data meta-analysis. *International Journal of Methods in Psychiatric Research*, *30*, e1860. https://doi.org/10.1002/mpr.1860

MacArthur, C., Winter, H. R., Bick, D. E., Knowles, H., Lilford, R., Henderson, C., Lancashire, R. J., Braunholtz, D. A., & Gee, H. (2002). Effects of redesigned community postnatal care on women's health 4 months after birth: A cluster randomized controlled trial. *Lancet*, *359*, 378–385.

Maes, M., Christophe, A., Bosmans, E., Lin, A., & Neels, H. (2000). In humans, serum polyunsaturated fatty acid levels predict the response of proinflammatory cytokines to psychologic stress. *Biological Psychiatry*, *47*, 910–920.

Maes, M., Yirmyia, R., Noraberg, J., Brene, S., Hibblen, J., Perini, G., Kubara, M., Bob, P., Lerer, B., & Maj, M. (2009). The inflammatory & neurodegenerative (I&ND) hypothesis of depression: Leads for future research and new drug development. *Metabolic Brain Disease*, *24*, 27–53.

Mahurin-Smith, J., & Beck, A. R. (2022). Self-compassion may protect against postpartum depression and anxiety. *Breastfeeding Review*, *30*(2), 27–34.

Maimburg, R. D., & Vaeth, M. (2015). Postpartum depression among first-time mothers – Results from a parallel randomised trial. *Sexual & Reproductive Healthcare*, *6*, 95–100.

Makrides, M., Gibson, R. A., & McPhee, A. J. (2010). Effect of DHA supplementation during pregnancy on maternal depression and neurodevelopment of young children: A randomized controlled trial. *JAMA*, *304*(15), 1675–1683.

Malm, H., Sourander, A., Gissler, M., Gyllenberg, D., Hinkka-Yli-Salomaki, S., McKeague, I. W., Artama, M., & Brown, A. S. (2015). Pregnancy complications following prenatal exposure to SSRIs or maternal psychiatric disorders: Results from population-based national register data. *American Journal of Psychiatry*, *172*, 1224–1232.

Manber, R., Schnyer, R. N., Allen, J. J. B., Rush, A. J., & Blasey, C. M. (2004). Acupuncture: A promising treatment for depression. *Journal of Affective Disorders*, *83*, 89–95.

Manber, R., Schnyer, R. N., Lyell, D., Chambers, A. S., Caughey, A. B., Druzin, M., Carlyle, E., Celio, C., Gress, J. L., Huang, M. I., Kalista, T., Martin-Okada, R., & Allen, J. J. B. (2010). Acupuncture for depression during pregnancy: A randomized controlled trial. *Obstetrics & Gynecology*, *115*(3), 511–520. https://doi.org/10.1097/AOG.0b013e3181cc0816

Mancini, F., Carlson, C., & Albers, L. (2007). Use of the Postpartum Depression Screening Scale in a collaborative obstetric practice. *Journal of Midwifery and Women's Health*, *52*(5), 429–434. https://doi.org/10.1016/j.jmwh.2007.03.007

Marangell, L. B., Martinez, J. M., Zboyan, H. A., Chong, H., & Puryear, L. J. (2004). Omega-3 fatty acids for the prevention of postpartum depression: Negative data from a preliminary, open-label pilot study. *Depression & Anxiety*, *19*, 20–23.

Marchesi, C. (2008). Pharmacological management of panic disorder. *Neuropsychiatric Disease and Treatment*, 4(1), 93–106.

Marchesi, C., Ossola, P., Amerio, A., Daniel, B. D., Tonna, M., & De Panfilis, C. (2016). Clinical management of perinatal anxiety disorders: A systematic review. *Journal of Affective Disorders*, 190, 543–550.

Marconcin, P., Peralta, M., Gouveia, E. R., Ferrari, G., Carraca, E., Ihle, A., & Marques, A. (2021). Effects of exercise during pregnancy on postpartum depression: A systematic review of meta-analyses. *Biology (Basel)*, 10(12), 1331. https://doi.org/10.3390/biology10121331

Markhus, M. W., Skotheim, S., Graff, I. E., Froyland, L., Braarud, H. C., Stormark, K. M., & Malde, M. K. (2013). Low omega-3 index in pregnancy is a possible biological risk factor for postpartum depression. *PLoS One*, 8, e67617. https://doi.org/10.1371/journal.pone.0067617

Markowitz, J. C., & Weissman, M. M. (2004). Interpersonal psychotherapy: Principles and applications. *World Psychiatry*, 3(3), 136–139.

Maschi, S., Clavenna, A., Campi, R., Schiavetti, B., Bernat, M., & Bonati, M. (2008). Neonatal outcome following pregnancy exposure to antidepressants: A prospective controlled cohort study. *British Journal of Obstetrics & Gynaecology*, 115, 283–289.

Matsumura, K., Hoguchi, H., Nishi, D., Hamazaki, K., Hamazaki, T., & Matsuoka, Y. J. (2017). Effects of omega-3 polyunsaturated fatty acids on psychophysiological symptoms of posttraumatic stress disorder in accident survivors: A randomized, double-blind, placebo-controlled trial. *Journal of Affective Disorders*, 224, 27–31.

Matthey, S., Lee, C., Crncec, R., & Trapolini, T. (2013). Errors in scoring the Edinburgh Postnatal Depression Scale. *Archives of Women's Mental Health*, 16, 117–122.

Maurer, D. M., Raymond, T. J., & Davis, B. N. (2018). Depression: Screening and diagnosis. *American Family Physician*, 98(8), 508–515.

McCarter-Spaulding, D., & Shea, S. (2016). Effectiveness of discharge education on postpartum depression. *MCN American Journal of Maternal-Child Nursing*, 41(3), 168–172. https://doi.org/10.1097/NMC.0000000000000236

McClellan, H. L., Hepworth, A. R., Garbin, C. P., Rowan, M. K., Deacon, J., Hartmann, P. E., & Geddes, D. T. (2012). Nipple pain during breastfeeding with or without visible trauma. *Journal of Human Lactation*, 28(4), 511–521.

McClintock, S. W., Reti, I. M., Carpenter, L. L., McDonald, W. M., Dubin, M., & Taylor, S. F. (2018). Consensus recommendations for the clinical application of repetitive transcranial magnetic stimulation (rTMS) in the treatment of depression. *Journal of Clinical Psychiatry*, 79(1), 16cs10905. https://doi.org/10.4088/JCP.16cs10905

McGarry, J., Kim, H., Sheng, X., Egger, M., & Baksh, L. (2009). Postpartum depression and help-seeking behavior. *Journal of Midwifery and Women's Health*, 54(1), 50–59.

McLeish, J., Ayers, S., & McCourt, C. (2023). Community-based perinatal mental health peer support: A realist review. *BMC Pregnancy and Childbirth*. https://doi.org/10.21203/rs.3.rs-2668499/v1

McNamara, R. K. (2009). Evaluation of docosahexaenoic acid deficiency as a preventable risk factor for recurrent affective disorders: Current status, future directions, and dietary recommendations. *Prostaglandins, Leukotrienes, and Essential Fatty Acids*, 81, 223–231.

McPhail, J., Loitz, C. C., Zaychkowsky, C., Valeroso, G., McNeil, D. A., McDonald, S. W., & Edwards, S. A. (2021). Opportunistic postpartum depression screening at well-child clinics in Alberta, 2012–2016. *Canadian Journal of Public Health*, 112, 938–946. https://doi.org/10.17269/s41997-021-00521-8

Meades, R., Pond, C., Ayers, S., & Warren, F. (2011). Postnatal debriefing: Have we thrown the baby out with the bath water? *Behavior Research and Therapy*, 49, 367–372.

Meltzer-Brody, S., Boschloo, L., Jones, I., Sullivan, P. F., & Penninx, B. W. (2013). The EPDS-Lifetime: Assessment of lifetime prevalence and risk factors for perinatal depression in a large cohort of depressed women. *Archives of Women's Mental Health*, 16, 465–473.

Menschner, C., & Maul, A. (2016). *Key ingredients for successful trauma-informed care implementation.* www.samhsa.gov/sites/default/files/programs_campaigns/childrens_mental_health/atc-whitepaper-040616.pdf

Middleton, P., Gomersall, J. C., Gould, J. F., Shepherd, E., Olsen, S. F., & Makrides, M. (2018). Omega-3 fatty acid addition during pregnancy. *Cochrane Database of Systematic Reviews, 11*(11), CD003402.

Milani, H. S., Amiri, P., Monfared, E. D., Vaziri, S. M., Malekkhah, A., & Salmani, F. (2017). Effect of health care as the "home visiting" on postpartum depression: A controlled clinical trial. *International Journal of Preventive Medicine, 8,* 20. https://doi.org/10.4103/2008-7802.204003

Milgrom, J., Gemmill, A. W., Ericksen, J., Burrows, G., Buist, A., & Reece, J. (2015). Treatment of postnatal depression with cognitive-behavioural therapy, sertraline, and combination therapy: A randomised controlled trial. *Australia New Zealand Journal of Psychiatry, 9*(3), 236–245. https://doi.org/10.1177/0004867414565474

Milgrom, J., Negri, L. M., Gemmill, A. W., McNeil, M., & Martin, P. R. (2005). A randomized controlled trial of psychological interventions for postnatal depression. *British Journal of Clinical Psychology, 44,* 529–542.

Miller, A. L. (2008). The methylation, neurotransmitter, and antioxidant connections between folate and depression. *Alternative Medicine Review, 13*(3), 216–225.

Miniati, M., Callari, A., Calugi, S., Rucci, P., Savino, M., Mauri, M., & Dell'Osso, L. (2014). Interpersonal psychotherapy for postpartum depression: A systematic review. *Archives of Women's Mental Health, 17,* 257–268.

Misri, S., Reebye, P., Corral, M., & Mills, L. (2004). The use of paroxetine and cognitive-behavioral therapy in postpartum depression and anxiety: A randomized controlled trial. *Journal of Clinical Psychiatry, 65,* 1236–1241.

Misri, S., Reebye, P., Milis, L., & Shah, S. (2006). The impact of treatment intervention on parenting stress in postpartum depressed women: A prospective study. *American Journal of Orthopsychiatry, 76*(1), 115–119.

Missler, M., van Straten, A., Denissen, J., Donker, T., & Beijers, R. (2020). Effectiveness of a psycho-educational intervention for expecting parents to prevent postpartum stress, depression, and anxiety: A randomized controlled trial. *BMC Pregnancy and Childbirth, 20,* 658. https://doi.org/10.1186/s12884-020-03341-9

Mitchell, J. E., Trangle, M., Degnan, B., Gabert, T. B., Haight, B., Kessler, D., & Mack, N. (2013). *Adult depression in primary care.* Institute for Clinical Systems Improvement.

Miyake, Y., Sasaki, S., Yokoyama, T., Tanaka, K., Ohya, Y., Fukushima, W., Saito, K., Ohfuji, S., Kiyohara, C., & Hirota, Y. (2006). Risk of postpartum depression in relation to dietary fish and fat intake in Japan: The Osaka Maternal and Child Health Study. *Psychological Medicine, 36,* 1727–1735.

Mocking, R. J. T., Steijn, K., Roos, C., Assies, J., Bergink, V., Ruhe, H. G., & Schene, A. H. (2020). Omega-3 fatty acid supplementation for perinatal depression: A meta-analysis. *Journal of Clinical Psychiatry, 81*(5), 19r13195. https://doi.org/10.4088/JCP.19r13106

Molero, P., Ramos-Quiroga, J. A., Martin-Santos, R., Calvo-Sanchez, E., Gutierrez-Rojas, L., & Meana, J. J. (2018). Antidepressant efficacy and tolerability of ketamine and esketamine: A critical review. *CNS Drugs, 32*(5), 411–420. https://doi.org/10.1007/s40263-018-0519-3

Mollayeva, T., Thurairajah, P., Burton, K., Mollayeva, S., Shapiro, C. M., & Colantonio, A. (2016). The Pittsburgh Sleep Quality Index as a screening tool for sleep dysfunction in clinical and non-clinical samples: A systematic review and meta-analysis. *Sleep Medicine Reviews, 25,* 52–73. https://doi.org/10.1016/j.smrv.2015.01.009

Mortensen, K., & Kam, R. (2012). Exercise and breastfeeding. *Breastfeeding Review, 20*(3), 39–42.

Moses-Kolko, E. L., & Roth, E. K. (2004). Antepartum and postpartum depression: Healthy mom, healthy baby. *Journal of the American Medical Women's Association, 59,* 181–191.

Moussa, S., Fawaz, L., Ibrahim, W., Elsayed, M. F., & Ahmed, M. M. (2021). Effect of infant massage on salivary oxytocin level of mothers and infants with normal and disordered bonding. *Journal of Primary Care and Community Health*, 12, 1–8. https://doi.org/10.1177/21501327211012942

Moyer, S. W., Kinser, P. A., Nunziato, J. D., Holmes, C. M., & Salisbury, A. L. (2023). Development of the Edinburgh Postnatal Depression Scale-United States: An updated perinatal mental health screening tool using a respectful care and trauma-informed approach. *Journal of Women's Health*. https://doi.org/10.1089/jwh.2023.0141

Mufson, L., Dorta, K. P., Wickramaratne, P., Nomura, Y., Olfson, M., & Weissman, M. M. (2004). A randomized effectiveness trial of interpersonal psychotherapy for depressed adolescents. *Archives of General Psychiatry*, 61, 577–584.

Muller, W. E. (2003). Current St. John's wort research from mode of action to clinical efficacy. *Pharmacology Research*, 47, 101–109.

Myers, E. R., Aubuchon-Endsley, N., Bastian, L. A., Gierisch, J. M., Kemper, A. R., & Swamy, G. K. (2013). *Efficacy and safety of screening for postpartum depression.* Agency for Healthcare Research and Quality.

National Alliance on Mental Illness (NAMI). (2007). *Seasonal affective disorder.* www.nami.org

National Center for PTSD. (2010). *Mindfulness practice in the treatment of traumatic stress.* www.ptsd.va.gov/public/pages/mindful-ptsd.asp

National Center for PTSD. (2014). *Treatment for PTSD.* www.ptsd.va.gov/public/treatment/therapy-med/treatment-ptsd.asp

National Center for PTSD. (2015). *Women, trauma and PTS.* www.ptsd.va.gov/public/ptsd-overview/women/women-trauma-and-ptsd.asp

National Health Service. (2022). *Treatment – posttraumatic stress disorder.* www.nhs.uk/mental-health/conditions/post-traumatic-stress-disorder-ptsd/treatment/

Newport, D. J., Hostetter, A., Arnold, A., & Stowe, Z. (2002). The treatment of postpartum depression: Minimizing infant exposures. *Journal of Clinical Psychiatry*, 63(Suppl 7), 31–44.

Nicolson, S., Judd, F., Thomson-Salo, F., & Mitchell, S. (2013). Supporting the adolescent mother-infant relationship: Preliminary trial of a brief perinatal attachment intervention. *Archives of Women's Mental Health*, 16, 511–520.

Nikayin, S., Murphy, E., Krystal, J. H., & Wilkinson, S. T. (2022). Long-term safety of ketamine and esktamine in treatment of depression. *Expert Opinion on Drug Safety*, 21(6), 777–787. https://doi.org/10.1080/14740338.2022.2066651

Noaghiul, S., & Hibbeln, J. R. (2003). Cross-national comparisons of seafood consumption and rates of bipolar disorders *American Journal of Psychiatry*, 160, 2222–2227.

Noorbakhshnia, M., Dehkordi, N. G., Ghaedi, K., Esmaeili, A., & Dabaghi, M. (2015). Omega-3 fatty acids prevent LPS-induced passive avoidance learning and memory and CaMKII-gene expression impairments in hippocampus of rat. *Pharmacological Reports*, 67, 370–375.

Norman, E., Sherburn, M., Osborne, R., & Galea, M. P. (2010). An exercise and education program improves well-being of new mothers: A randomized controlled trial. *Physical Therapy*, 90, 348–355.

Nutor, J. J., Slaughter-Acey, J. C., Giurgescu, C., & Misra, D. P. (2018). Symptoms of depression and preterm birth among Black women. *MCN American Journal of Maternal-Child Nursing*, 43(5), 252–258. https://doi.org/10.1097/NMC.0000000000000464

Nylen, K. J., O'Hara, M. W., Brock, R., Moel, J., Gorman, L., & Stuart, S. (2010). Predictors of the longitudinal course of postpartum depression following interpersonal psychotherapy. *Journal of Consulting & Clinical Psychology*, 78, 757–763.

Oberlander, T. F., Reebye, P., Misri, S., Papsdorf, M., Kim, J., & Grunau, R. E. (2007). Externalizing and attentional behaviors in children of depressed mothers treated with selective-serotonin reuptake inhibitor antidepressant during pregnancy. *Archives of Pediatric & Adolescent Medicine*, 161, 22–29.

Oberlander, T. F., Warburton, W., Misri, S., Aghajanian, J., & Hertzman, C. (2006). Neonatal outcome after prenatal exposure to selective-serotonin reuptake inhibitor antidepressants and maternal depression using population-based linked health data. *Archives of Women's Mental Health*, *63*, 898–906.

O'Brien, S. M., Scott, L. V., & Dinan, T. G. (2006). Antidepressant therapy and C-reactive protein levels. *British Journal of Psychiatry*, *188*, 449–452. https://doi.org/10.1192/bjp.bp.105.011015

O'Connor, E., Rossom, R. C., Henniger, M., Groom, H. C., & Burda, B. U. (2016). Primary care screening for and treatment of depression in pregnant and postpartum women: Evidence report and systematic review for the US Preventive Services Task Force. *JAMA*, *315*(41), 388–406.

O'Hara, M. W. (2022). Peer-delivered psychotherapy for postpartum depression: Has its time come? *Journal of Clinical Psychiatry*, *81*(1). https://doi.org/10.4088/JCP.21m13928

O'Hara, M. W., & Engeldinger, J. (2018). Treatment of postpartum depression: Recommendations for the clinician. *Clinical Obstetrics & Gynecology*, *61*(3), 604–614.

O'Hara, M. W., Pearlstein, T., Stuart, S., Long, J. D., Mills, J. A., & Zlotnick, C. (2019). A placebo controlled treatment trial of sertraline and interpersonal psychotherapy for postpartum depression. *Journal of Affective Disorders*, *245*, 524–532. https://doi.org/10.1016/j.jad.2018.10.361

O'Hara, M. W., Stuart, S., Gorman, L. L., & Wenzel, A. (2000). Efficacy of interpersonal psychotherapy for postpartum depression. *Archives of General Psychiatry*, *57*, 1039–1045.

Olafsdottir, A. S., Skuladottir, G. V., Thorsdottir, I., Hauksson, A., Thorgeirsdottir, H., & Steingrimsdottir, L. (2006). Relationship between high consumption of marine fatty acids in early pregnancy and hypertensive disorders in pregnancy. *British Journal of Obstetrics & Gynecology*, *113*, 301–309.

Olin, S.-C. S., Kerker, B. D., Stein, R. E. K., Weiss, D., Whitmyre, E. D., Hoagwood, K. E., & Horwitz, S. M. (2016). Can postpartum depression be managed in pediatric primary care? *Journal of Women's Health*, *25*(4), 381–389. https://doi.org/10.1089/jwh.2015.5438

Onozawa, K., Glover, V., Adams, D., Modi, N., & Kumar, R. C. (2001). Infant massage improves mother-infant interaction for mothers with postnatal depression. *Journal of Affective Disorders*, *63*, 201–207.

Oren, D. A., Wisner, K. L., Spinelli, M., Epperson, C. N., Peindl, K. S., Terman, J. S., & Terman, M. (2002). An open trial of morning light therapy for treatment of antepartum depression. *American Journal of Psychiatry*, *159*, 666–669.

Orhon, F. S., Ulukol, B., & Soykan, A. (2007). Postpartum mood disorders and maternal perceptions of infant patterns in well-child follow-up visits. *Acta Paediatrica*, *96*, 1777–1783.

Osborne, L., Birndorf, C. A., Szkodny, L. E., & Wisner, K. L. (2014). Returning to tricyclic antidepressants for depression during childbearing: Clinical and dosing challenges. *Archives of Women's Mental Health*, *17*, 239–246.

Osorio, F. d. L., Darwin, A. C. R., Bombonetti, E. A., & Ayers, S. (2022). Posttraumatic stress following childbirth: Psychometric properties of the Brazilian version of the City Birth Trauma Scale. *Journal of Psychosomatic Obstetrics & Gynecology*, *43*(3), 374–383. https://doi.org/10.1080/0167482X.2021.1977278

Pace, T. W., Hu, F., & Miller, A. H. (2007). Cytokine-effects on glucocorticoid receptor function: Relevance to glucocorticoid resistance and the pathophysiology and treatment of major depression. *Brain, Behavior and Immunity*, *21*(1), 9–19. https://doi.org/10.1016/j.bbi.2006.08.009

Peeler, S., Chung, M. C., Stedmon, J., & Skirton, H. (2012). A review assessing current treatment strategies for postnatal psychological morbidity with a focus on post-traumatic stress disorder. *Midwifery*. https://doi.org/10.1016/j.midw.2012.03.004

Penckofer, S., Kouba, J., Wallis, D. E., & Emanuele, M. A. (2008). Vitamin D and diabetes. *Nutrition Update*, *34*, 939–954.

Peng, L., Fu, C., Xiong, F., Zhang, Q., Liang, Z., Chen, L., He, C., & Wei, Q. (2020). Effects of repetitive transcranial magnetic stimulation on depression symptoms and cognitive function in treating patients with postpartum depression: A systematic review and meta-analysis of randomized controlled trials. *Psychiatric Research*, *290*. https://doi.org/10.1016/j.psychres.2020.113124

Peng, Y., Ao, M., Dong, B., Jiang, Y., Yu, L., Chen, Z., Hu, C., & Xu, R. (2021). Anti-inflammatory effects of curcumin in the inflammatory diseases: Status, limitations, and countermeasures. *Drug Design, Development and Therapy*, 15, 4503–4525. https://doi.org/10.2147/DDDT.S327378

Pennebaker, J. (2004). *Writing to heal: A guided journal for recovering from trauma and emotional upheaval* Center for Journal Therapy.

Pereira, A. T., Bos, S., Marques, M., Maia, B. R., Soares, M. J., Valente, J., Gomes, A. A., Macedo, A., & de Azevedo, M. H. P. (2011). The postpartum depression screening scale: Is it valid to screen for antenatal depression? *Archives of Women's Mental Health*, 14(3), 227–238. https://doi.org/10.1007/s00737-010-0178-y

Perez-Blasco, J., Viguer, P., & Rodrigo, M. F. (2013). Effects of a mindfulness-based intervention on psychological distress, well-being, and maternal self-efficacy in breastfeeding mothers: Results of a pilot study. *Archives of Women's Mental Health*, 16, 227–236.

Porter, L. S., Porter, B. O., McCoy, V., Bango-Sanchez, V., Kissel, B., Williams, M., & Nunnewar, S. (2015). Blended infant massage-parenting enhancement program on recovering substance-abusing mothers' parenting stress, self-esteem, depression, maternal attachment, and mother-infant interaction. *Asian Nursing Research*, 9, 318–327. http://dx.doi.org/10.1016/j.anr.2015.09.002

Poyatos-Leon, R., Garcia-Hermoso, A., Sanabria-Martinez, G., Alvarez-Bueno, C., Cavero-Redondo, I., & Martinez-Vizcaino, V. (2017). Effects of exercise-based interventions on postpartum depression: A meta-analysis of randomized controlled trials. *Birth*, 44, 200–208. https://doi.org/10.1111/birt.12294

Preston, J., Moore, B. A., & Johnson, J. (2022). *Clinical psychopharmacology made ridiculously simple*. Medmaster.

Pritchett, R. V., Jolly, K., Turner, K., Sharp, D., Bradbury-Jones, C., Daley, A. J., & PAM-PeRS Study. (2017). Women's views of exercise as a treatment for postnatal depression: A qualitative study. *Journal of Health Psychology*, http://doi.org/10.1177/1359105317726590.

Qui, C., Gelaye, B., Zhong, Q., Enquobahrie, D. A., Frederick, I. O., & Williams, M. A. (2016). Construct validity and factor structure of the Pittsburgh Sleep Quality Index among pregnant women in a Pacific-Northwest cohort. *Sleep & Breathing*, 20(1), 293–301. https://doi.org/10.1007/s11325-016-1313-4

Quinn, T. J., & Carey, G. B. (1999). Does exercise intensity or diet influence lactic acid accumulation in breast milk? *Medicine and Science in Sports and Exercise*, 31, 105–110.

Rados, S. N., Matijas, M., Kuhar, L., Andelinovic, M., & Ayers, S. (2020). Measuring and conceptualizing PTSD following childbirth: Validation of the City Birth Trauma Scale. *Psychological Trauma*, 12(2), 147–155. https://doi.org/10.1037/tra0000501

Rados, S. N., Tadinac, M., & Herman, R. (2018). Anxiety during pregnancy and postpartum course: Predictors and comorbidity with postpartum depression. *Acta Clinica Croatia*, 57, 39–51. https://doi.org/10.20471/acc.2018.57.01.05

Rafferty, J., Mattson, G., Earls, M. F., Yogman, M. W., Gambon, T. B., Lavin, A., & Wissow, L. S. (2019). Incorporating recognition and management of perinatal depression into pediatric practice. *Pediatrics*, 143(1), e20183260. https://doi.org/10.1542/peds.2018-3260

Rahmatnezhad, L., Sheikhi, S., Didarloo, A., Fakoor, Z., & Iranidokht, M. (2018). The impact of baby massage training on awareness, perceived stress, and breastfeeding self-efficacy of mothers with hospitalized neonates. *International Journal of Pediatrics*, 6(10), 8297–8306. https://doi.org/10.22038/ijp.2018.32043.2833

Ramakrishna, S., Cooklin, A. R., & Leach, L. S. (2019). Comorbid anxiety and depression: A community-based study examining symptomology and correlates during the postpartum period. *Journal of Reproductive and Infant Psychology*, 37, 468–479. https://doi.org/10.1080/02646838.2019.1578870

Rampono, J., Teoh, S., Hackett, L. P., Kohan, R., & Illet, K. F. (2011). Estimation of desvenlafaxine transfer into milk and infant exposure during its use in lactating women with postnatal depression. *Archives of Women's Mental Health*, 14, 49–53.

Reay, R. E., Owen, C., Shadbolt, B., Raphael, B., Mulcahy, R., & Wilkinson, R. B. (2012). Trajectories of long-term outcomes for postnatally depressed mothers treated with group interpersonal psychotherapy. *Archives of Women's Mental Health, 15,* 217–228.

Rechenberg, K., & Humphries, D. (2013). Nutritional intervention is in depression and perinatal depression. *Yale Journal of Biology and Medicine, 66,* 127–137.

Rees, A.-M., Austin, M.-P., & Parker, G. (2005). Role of omega-3 fatty acids as a treatment for depression in the perinatal period. *Australia & New Zealand Journal of Psychiatry, 39,* 274–280.

Reid, K. M., & Taylor, M. G. (2015). Social support, stress, and maternal postpartum depression: A comparison of supportive relationships. *Social Science & Medicine, 54,* 246–262.

Reza, N., Deligiannidis, K. M., Eustis, E. H., & Battle, C. L. (2018). Complementary health practices for treating perinatal depression. *Obstetrics & Gynecology Clinics, 45*(3), 441–454.

Robertson-Blackmore, E., Putnam, F. W., Rubinow, D. R., Matthieu, M., Hunn, J. E., Putnam, K. T., Moynihan, J., & O'Connor, T. G. (2013). Antecedent trauma exposure and risk of depression in the perinatal period. *Journal of Clinical Psychiatry, 74*(10), e942–e948.

Robinson, M., Whitehouse, A. J. O., Newnham, J. P., Gorman, S., Jacoby, P., Holt, B. J., Serralha, M., Tearne, J. E., Holt, P. G., Hart, P. H., & Kusel, M. M. H. (2014). Low maternal serum vitamin D during pregnancy and the risk for postpartum depression symptoms. *Archive of Women's Mental Health, 17*(3), 213–219. https://doi.org/10.1007/s00737-014-0422-y

Rodriguez-Munoz, M. D. L. F., Ruiz-Segovia, N., Soto-Balbuena, C., Le, H.-N., Olivares-Crespo, M. E., & Izquierdo-Mendez, N. (2020). The psychometric properties of the Patient Health Questionnaire-4 for pregnant women. *International Journal of Environmental Research in Public Health, 17,* 7583. https://doi.org/10.3390/ijerph17207583

Romieu, I., Torrent, M., Garcia-Esteban, R., Ferrer, C., Ribas-Fito, N., Anto, J. M., & Sunyer, J. (2007). Maternal fish intake during pregnancy and atopy and asthma in infancy. *Clinical & Experimental Allergy, 37,* 518–525.

Roubenoff, R. (2003). Exercise and inflammatory disease. *Arthritis Care & Research, 49*(2), 263–266.

Roumestan, C., Michel, A., Bichon, F., Portet, K., Detoc, M., Henriquet, C., Jaffuel, D., & Mathieu, M. (2007). Anti-inflammatory properties of desipramine and fluoxetine. *Respiratory Research, 8,* 35. https://doi.org/10.1186/1465-9921-8-35

Rowan, P. J., Duckett, S. A., & Wang, J. E. (2015). State mandates regarding postpartum depression. *Psychiatric Services, 66*(3), 324–328.

Rupke, S. J., Blecke, D., & Renfrow, M. (2006). Cognitive therapy for depression. *American Family Physician, 73,* 83–86.

Sandoz, V., Hingray, C., Stuijfzand, S., Lacroix, A., El Hage, W., & Horsch, A. (2022). Measurement and conceptualization of the Maternal PTSD following childbirth: Psychometric properties of the City Birth Trauma Scale – French version (City BiTS-F). *Psychological Trauma, 14*(4), 696–704. https://doi.org/10.1037/tra0001068

Sangsawang, B., Wacharasin, C., & Sangsawang, N. (2019). Interventions for the prevention of postpartum depression in adolescent mothers: A systematic review. *Archives of Women's Mental Health, 22,* 215–228. https://doi.org/10.1007/s00737-018-0901-7

Santucci, A. K., Singer, L. T., Wisniewski, S., Luther, J. F., Eng, H. F., Dills, J. L., & Sit, D. K. (2014). Impact of prenatal exposure to serotonin reuptake inhibitors or maternal major depressive disorder on infant developmental outcomes. *Journal of Clinical Psychiatry, 75,* 1088–1095.

Schultz, V. (2006). Safety of St. John's wort extract compared to synthetic antidepressants. *Phytomedicine, 13,* 199–204.

Seghete, K. L. M., Graham, A. M., Lapidus, J. A., Jackson, E. L. A., Doyle, O. J., Feryn, A. B., Moore, L. A., Goodman, S. H., & Dimidjian, S. (2020). Protocol for a mechanistic study of mindfulness-based cognitive therapy during pregnancy. *Health Psychology, 39*(9), 758–766. http://dx.doi.org/10.1037/hea0000870

Sharma, V., & Xie, B. (2011). Screening for postpartum bipolar disorder: Validation of the Mood Disorder Questionnaire. *Journal of Affective Disorders, 131*(1–3), 408–411. https://doi.org/10.1016/j.jad.2010.11.026

Shaw, R. J., St. John, N., Lilo, E., Jo, B., Benitz, W., Stevenson, D. K., & Horwitz, S. M. (2014). Prevention of traumatic stress in mothers of preterms: 6-month outcomes. *Pediatrics, 134*(2), e481–e488.

Shitu, S., Geda, B., & Dheresa, M. (2019). Postpartum depression and associated factors among mothers who gave birth in the last twelve months in Ankesha district, Awi zone, North West Ethiopia. *BMC Pregnancy and Childbirth, 19*, 435. https://doi.org/10.1186/s12884-019-2594-y

Shoji, H., Franke, C., Campoy, C., Rivero, M., Demmelmair, H., & Koletzko, B. (2006). Effect of docosahexaenoic acid and eicosapentaenoic acid supplementation on oxidative stress levels during pregnancy. *Free Radical Research, 40*, 379–384.

Shrestha, S. D., Pradhan, R., Tran, T. D., Gualano, R. C., & Fisher, J. R. W. (2016). Reliability and validity of the Edinburgh Postnatal Depression Scale (EPDS) for detecting perinatal common mental disorders (PCMDs) among women in low-and lower-middle-income countries: A systematic review. *BMC Pregnancy and Childbirth, 16*, http://doi.org/10.1186/S12884-019-2584-y

Shulman, B., Dueck, R., Ryan, D., Breau, G., Sadowski, I., & Misri, S. (2018). Feasibility of a mindfulness-based cognitive therapy group intervention as an adjunctive treatment for postpartum depression and anxiety. *Journal of Affective Disorders, 235*, 61–67. https://doi.org/10.1016/j.jad.2017.12.065

Sidebottom, A. C., Harrison, P. A., Godecker, A., & Kim, H. (2012). Validation of the Patient Health Questionnaire (PHQ)-9 for prenatal depression screening. *Archives of Women's Mental Health, 12*, 367–374.

Sigurdardottir, S., & Halldorsdottir, S. (2018). Screaming body and silent healthcare providers: A case study with a childhood sexual abuse (CSA) survivor. *International Journal of Environmental Research in Public Health, 15*, 94. https://doi.org/10.3390/ijerph15010094

Simpson, M., & Catling, C. (2016). Understanding psychological traumatic birth: A literature review. *Women & Birth, 29*, 203–207.

Siu, A. L., & US Preventive Services Task Force (USPSTF). (2016). Screening for depression in adults: US Preventive Services Task Force recommendations. *JAMA, 315*(4), 380–387. https://doi.org/10.1001/jama.2015.18392

Skurtveit, S., Selmer, R., Roth, C., Hernandez-Diaz, S., & Handal, M. (2014). Prenatal exposure to antidepressants and language competence at age three: Results from a large population-based pregnancy cohort in Norway. *British Journal of Obstetrics & Gynaecology, 121*, 1621–1631. https://doi.org/10.1111/1471-0528.12821

Slavin, V., Creedy, D. K., & Gamble, J. (2020). Comparison of screening accuracy of the Patient Health Questionnaire-2 using two case-identification methods during pregnancy and postpartum. *BMC Pregnancy and Childbirth, 20*, 211. https://doi.org/10.1186/s12884-020-02891-2

Small, R., Lumley, J., Donohue, L., Potter, A., & Waldenstrom, U. (2000). Randomised controlled trial of midwife-led debriefing to reduce maternal depression after operative childbirth. *British Medical Journal, 321*, 1043–1047.

Smith-Apeldoorn, S. Y., Ke Veraart, J., Spijker, J., Kamphuis, J., & Schoevers, R. A. (2022). Maintenance ketamine treatment for depression: A systematic review of efficacy, safety, and tolerability. *Lancet Psychiatry, 9*(11), 907–921. https://doi.org/10.1016/S2215-0366(22)00317-0

Smith-Nielsen, J., Matthey, S., Lange, T., & Vaever, M. S. (2018). Validation of the Edinburgh Postnatal Depression Scale against both DSM-5 and ICD-10 diagnostic criteria for depression. *BMC Psychiatry, 18*, 393. https://doi.org/10.1186/s12888-018-1965-7

Smuts, C. M., Huang, M., Mundy, D., Plasse, T., Major, S., & Carlson, S. E. (2003). A randomized trial of docosahexaenoic acid supplementation during the third trimester of pregnancy. *Obstetrics & Gynecology, 101*, 469–479.

Sockol, L. E., Epperson, C. N., & Barber, J. P. (2013). Preventing postpartum depression: A meta-analytic review. *Clinical Psychological Review, 33*(8), 1205–1217. https://doi.org/10.1016/j.cpr.2013.10.004

Speisman, B. B., Storch, E. A., & Abramowitz, J. S. (2011). Postpartum obsessive-compulsive disorder. *Journal of Obstetric, Gynecologic, and Neonatal Nursing, 40,* 680–690.

Spinelli, M. G., & Endicott, J. (2003). Controlled clinical trial of interpersonal psychotherapy versus parenting education program for depressed pregnant women. *American Journal of Psychiatry, 160,* 555–562.

Staneva, A., Bogossian, F., Pritchard, M., & Wittkowski, A. (2015). The effects of maternal depression, anxiety, and perceived stress during pregnancy on preterm birth: A systematic review. *Women & Birth, 28*(3), 179–193. https://doi.org/10.1016/j.wombi.2015.02.003

Starcevic, V., Eslick, G. D., Viswasam, K., & Berle, D. (2020). Symptoms of obsessive-compulsive disorder during pregnancy and the postpartum period: A systematic review and meta-analysis. *Psychiatric Quarterly, 91*(4). https://doi.org/10.1007/s11126-020-09769-8

Starkweather, A. R. (2007). The effects of exercise on perceived stress and IL-6 levels among older adults. *Biological Research for Nursing, 8,* 1–9.

Statistics Canada. (2019). Maternal mental health in Canada, 2018/2019. *The Daily.* https://www150.statcan.gc.ca/n1/daily-quotidien/190624/dq190624b-eng.htm

Sten, G., Ayers, S., Malquist, A., Nieminen, K., & Grundstrom, H. (2023). Assessment of maternal posttraumatic stress disorder following childbirth: Psychometric properties of the Swedish version of the City Birth Trauma Scale. *Psychological Trauma.* https://doi.org/10.1037/tra0001465

Stern, G., & Kruckman, L. (1983). Multi-disciplinary perspectives on postpartum depression: An anthropological critique. *Social Science & Medicine, 17,* 1027–1041.

Stewart, D. E., & Vigod, S. N. (2019). Postpartum depression: Pathophysiology, treatment, and emerging therapeutics. *Annual Review of Medicine, 70,* 181–196. https://doi.org/10.1146/annurev-med-041217-011106

Stramrood, C. A., van der Velde, J., Doornbos, B., Paarlberg, K. M., Weijmar Schultz, W. C. M., & Van Pampus, M. G. (2012). The patient observer: Eye-movement desensitization and reprocessing for the treatment of posttraumatic stress following childbirth. *Birth, 39*(1), 70–76.

Su, D., Zhao, Y., Binna, C., Scott, J., & Oddy, W. (2007). Breast-feeding mothers can exercise: Results of a cohort study. *Public Health Nutrition, 10,* 1089–1093.

Su, K.-P., Huang, S.-Y., Chiu, T.-H., Huang, K.-C., Huang, C.-L., Chang, H.-C., & Pariante, C. M. (2008). Omega-3 fatty acids for major depressive disorder during pregnancy: Results from a randomized, double-blind, placebo trial. *Journal of Clinical Psychiatry, 69,* 644–651.

Suarez, E. C. (2006). Sex differences in the relation of depressive symptoms, hostility, and anger expression to indices of glucose metabolism in nondiabetic adults. *Health Psychology, 25,* 484–492.

Suarez, E. C., Lewis, J. G., Krishnan, R. R., & Young, K. H. (2004). Enhanced expression of cytokines and chemokines by blood monocytes to in vitro lipopolysaccharide stimulation are associated with hostility and severity of depressive symptoms in healthy women. *Psychoneuroendocrinology, 29,* 1119–1128.

Substance Abuse and Mental Health Services Administration (SAMHSA). (2015). *Trauma-informed approach and trauma-specific interventions.* U.S. Government Printing Office. http://www.samhsa.gov/nctic/trauma-interventions

Sullivan, B., & Payne, T. W. (2007). Affective disorders and cognitive failures: A comparison of seasonal and nonseasonal depression. *American Journal of Psychiatry, 164,* 1663–1667.

Sun, Y., Fu, Z., Bo, Q., Mao, Z., Ma, X., & Wang, C. (2020). The reliability and validity of PHQ-9 in patients with major depressive disorder in psychiatric hospitals. *BMC Psychiatry, 20,* 474. http://doi.org/10.1186/s12888-020-02885-6

Swalm, D., Brooks, J., Doherty, D., Nathan, E., & Jacques, A. (2010). Using the Edinburgh Postnatal Depression Scale to screen for perinatal anxiety. *Archives of Women's Mental Health, 13,* 515–522.

Sword, W., Busser, D., Ganann, R., McMillan, T., & Swinton, M. (2008). Women's care-seeking experiences after referral for postpartum depression. *Qualitative Health Research, 18*(9), 1161–1173.

Szajewska, H., Horvath, A., & Koletzko, B. (2006). Effect of n-3 long-chain polyunsaturated fatty acid supplementation of women with low-risk pregnancies on pregnancy outcomes and growth measures at birth: A meta-analysis of randomized controlled trials. *American Journal of Clinical Nutrition, 83*, 1337–1344.

Szegedi, A., Kohnen, R., Dienel, A., & Kieser, M. (2005). Acute treatment of moderate to severe depression with hypericum extract WS 5570 (St. John's wort): Randomised controlled double blind non-inferiority trial versus paroxetine. *British Medical Journal, 330*, 503. https://doi.org/10.1136/bmj.38356.655266.82

Terman, M., & Terman, J. S. (2005). Light therapy for seasonal and nonseasonal depression: Efficacy, protocol, safety, and side effects. *CNS Spectrums, 10*, 647–663.

Terman, M., & Terman, J. S. (2006). Controlled trial of naturalistic dawn simulation and negative air ionization for seasonal affective disorder. *American Journal of Psychiatry, 163*, 2126.

Teychenne, M., & York, R. (2013). Physical activity, sedentary behavior, and postnatal depressive symptoms: A review. *American Journal of Preventive Medicine, 45*, 217–227.

Tong, P., Dong, L.-P., Yang, Y., Shi, Y.-H., Sun, T., & Bo, P. (2019). Traditional Chines acupuncture and postpartum depression: A systematic review and meta-analysis. *Journal of the Chinese Medical Association, 82*, 719–726. https://doi.org/10.1097/JCMA.0000000000000140

Uchino, B. N., Trettevik, R., Kent de Grey, R. G., Cronan, S., Hogan, J., & Baucom, B. R. W. (2018). Social support, social integration, and inflammatory cytokines: A meta-analysis. *Health Psychology, 37*(5), 462–471.

Uvnas-Moberg, K. (2015). *Oxytocin: The biological guide to motherhood*. Praeclarus Press.

VA/DoD Clinical Practice Guideline. (2023). *Management of posttraumatic stress disorders and acute stress disorder work group*. https://www.healthquality.va.gov/guidelines/MH/ptsd/

van der Kolk, B. A. (2002). Assessment and treatment of complex PTSD. In R. Yehuda (Ed.), *Treating trauma survivors with PTSD* (pp. 127–156). American Psychiatric Association Press.

Van Gurp, G., Meterissian, G. B., Haiek, L. N., McCusker, J., & Bellavance, F. (2002). St. John's wort or sertraline?: Randomized controlled trial in primary care. *Canadian Family Physician, 48*, 905–912.

Vogeli, J. M., Hooker, S. A., Everhart, K. D., & Kaplan, P. S. (2018). Psychometric properties of the postpartum depression screening scale beyond the postpartum period. *Research in Nursing & Health, 41*(2), 185–194. https://doi.org/10.1002/nur.21861

Volkow, N. D. (2019). Foreword. In I. D. Montoya & S. R. B. Weiss (Eds.), *Cannabis use disorder* (pp. v–vi). Springer Nature. https://doi.org/10.1007/978-3-319-90365-1

Vollmar, P., Haghikia, A., Dermietzel, R., & Faustmann, P. M. (2008). Venlafaxine exhibits an anti-inflammatory effect in an inflammatory co-culture model. *International Journal of Neuropsychopharmacology, 11*(1), 111–117. https://doi.org/10.1017/S1461145707007729

Wagner, C. L. (2011). Vitamin D: Recommendations during pregnancy, lactation, and early infancy. *Clinical Lactation, 2*(1), 27–31.

Wagner, C. L., Hulsey, T. C., Fanning, D., Ebeling, M., & Hollin, B. W. (2006). High dose vitamin D3 supplementation in a cohort of breastfeeding mothers and their infants. *Breastfeeding Medicine, 1*(2), 59–70.

Wagner, C. L., Taylor, S. N., & Hollis, B. (2010). *New insights into Vitamin D during pregnancy, lactation, and early infancy*. Praeclarus Press

Walker, E. R., Gao, J., & Xie, B. (2015). Postpartum psychosocial and behavioral health: A systematic review of self-administered scales validated for postpartum women in the United States. *Women's Health Issues, 25*, 586–600.

Walkery, A., Leader, L. D., Cooke, E., & VandenBerg, A. (2021). Review of allopregnanolone agonist therapy for the treatment of depressive disorders. *Drug Design, Development and Therapy, 15*, 3017–3026. https://doi.org/10.2147/DDDT.S240856

Wang, C., Chung, M., Lichtenstein, A., Balk, E., Kupelnick, B., DeVine, D., Lawrence, A., & Lau, J. (2004). *Effects of omega-3 fatty acids on cardiovascular disease* (Vol. AHRQ Publication No. 04-E009-1). Agency for Healthcare Research and Quality.

Wang, J., Luo, H., Schulke, R., Geng, X., Sahakian, B. J., & Wang, S. (2021). Is transcranial direct current stimulation, alone or in combination with antidepressant medications or psychotherapies, effective in treating major depressive disorder? A systematic review and meta-analysis. *BMC Medicine, 19*(1). https://doi.org/10.1186/s12916-021-02181-4

Wang, Y., Hu, Y.-P., Wang, W.-C., Pang, R.-Z., & Zhang, A.-R. (2012). Clinical studies on treatment of earthquake-caused posttraumatic stress disorder using electroacupuncture. *Evidence-Based Complementary and Alternative Medicine, 2012*(4), 431279. https://doi.org/10.1155/2012/431279

Wang, Y., Zhong, W., Zhao, A., Szeto, I. M.-Y., Lan, H., Zhang, J., Li, P., Ren, Z., Mao, S., Jiang, H., Wang, P., & Zhang, Y. (2023). Perinatal depression and serum vitamin D status: A cross-sectional study in urban China. *Journal of Affective Disorders, 322*, 214–220. https://doi.org/10.1016/j.jad.2022.11.030

Waqas, A., Malik, A., Atif, N., Nisar, A., Nazir, H., Sikander, S., & Rahman, A. (2021). Scalable screening and treatment response monitoring for perinatal depression in low- and middle-income countries. *International Journal of Environmental Research and Public Health, 18*(13), 6693. https://doi.org/10.3390/ijerph18136693

Weathers, F. W., Litz, B. T., Keane, T. M., Palmieri, P. A., Marx, B. P., & Schnurr, P. P. (2013). *PTSD checklist for DSM-5 (PCL-5)*. www.ptsd.va.gov/

Webb, R., Smith, A. M., Ayers, S., Wright, D. B., & Thornton, A. (2021). Development and validation of a measure of birth-related PTSD for fathers and birth partners: The City Birth Trauma Scale (Partner Version). *Frontiers in Psychology, 12*, 506779. https://doi.org/10.3389/fpsyg.2021.596779

Weigl, T., Beck-Hiestermann, F. M. L., Stenzel, N. M., Benson, S., Schedlowski, M., & Garthus-Niegel, S. (2021). Assessment of childbirth-related PTSD: Psychometric properties of the German version of the City Birth Trauma Scale. *Frontiers in Psychiatry, 12*, 731537. https://doi.org/10.3389/fpsyt.2021.731537

Weissman, M. M. (2007). Recent non-medication trials of interpersonal psychotherapy for depression. *International Journal of Neuropsychopharmacology, 10*, 117–122.

Werneke, U., Turner, T., & Priebe, S. (2006). Complementary medicines in psychiatry: Review of effectiveness and safety. *British Journal of Psychiatry, 188*, 109–121.

Wicke, F. S., Krakau, L., Lowe, B., Beutel, M. E., & Brahler, E. (2022). Update of the standardization of the Patient Health Questionnaire-4 (PHQ-4) in the general population. *Journal of Affective Disorders, 312*, 310–314. https://doi.org/10.1016/j.jad.2022.06.054

Williams, J. W., Gierisch, J. M., McDuffie, J., Strauss, J. L., & Nagi, A. (2011). *An overview of complementary and alternative medicine therapies for anxiety and depressive disorders: Supplement to efficacy of complementary and alternative medicine therapies for posttraumatic stress disorder*. Health Service Research & Development Service.

Williams, K. E., & Koleva, H. (2018). Identification and treatment of peripartum anxiety disorders. *Obstetric & Gynecology Clinics, 45*(3), 469–481.

Wirz-Justice, A., Bader, A., Frisch, U., Stieglitz, R.-D., Alder, J., & Bitzer, J. (2017). A randomized, double-blind, placebo-controlled study of light therapy for antepartum depression. *Journal of Clinical Psychiatry, 72*(7), 986–993.

Wisner, K. L., Logsdon, M. C., & Shanahan, B. R. (2008). Web-based education for postpartum depression: Conceptual development and impact. *Archives of Women's Mental Health, 11*(5–6), 377–385. http://www.doi.org/10.1007/s00737-008-0030-9

Wisner, K. L., Sit, D. K. Y., Hanusa, B. H., Moses-Kolko, E. L., Bogen, D. L., Hunker, D. F., Perel, J. M., Jones-Ivy, S., Bodner, L. M., & Singer, L. T. (2009). Major depression and antidepressant treatment: Impact of pregnancy and neonatal outcomes. *American Journal of Psychiatry, 166*, 557–566.

Wisner, K. L., Sit, D. K. Y., McShea, M., Luther, J. F., Eng, H. F., Dills, J. L., Moses-Kolko, E. L., & Wisniewski, S. (2017). Telephone-based depression care management for postpartum women: A randomized controlled trial. *Journal of Clinical Psychiatry, 78*(9), 1369–1375. https://doi.org/10.4088/JCP.15m10563

Woelk, H. (2000). Comparison of St. John's wort and imipramine for treating depression: Randomised controlled trial. *British Medical Journal, 321*, 536–539.

Wojcicki, J. M., & Heyman, M. B. (2011). Maternal omega-3 fatty acid supplementation and risk for perinatal maternal depression. *Journal of Maternal-Fetal & Neonatal Medicine, 24*(5), 680–686. https://doi.org/10.3109/14767058.2010.521873

World Health Organization. (2014). *The prevention and elimination of disrespect and abuse during facility-based childbirth.* http://apps.who.int/iris/bitstream/10665/134588/1/WHO_RHR_14.23_eng.pdf?ua=1&ua=1

Wurglies, M., & Schubert-Zsilavecz, M. (2006). Hypericum perforatum: A "modern" herbal antidepressant: Pharmacokinetics of active ingredients. *Clinical Pharmacokinetics, 45*, 449–468.

Yang, L., Di, Y. M., Shergis, J. L., Li, Y., Zhang, A. L., Lu, C., Guo, X., & Xue, C. C. (2018). A systematic review of acupuncture and Chinese herbal medicine for postpartum depression. *Complementary Therapies in Clinical Practice, 33*, 85–92. https://doi.org/10.1016/j.ctcp.2018.08.006

Yang, Y., Li, W., Ma, T.-J., Zhang, L., Hall, B. J., Ungvari, G. S., & Xiang, Y.-T. (2020). Prevalence of poor sleep quality in perinatal and postnatal women: A comprehensive meta-analysis of observational studies. *Frontiers in Psychiatry, 11*, 161. https://doi.org/10.3389/fpsyt.2020.00161

Yeaton-Massey, A., & Herrero, T. (2019). Recognizing maternal mental health disorders: Beyond postpartum depression. *Current Opinions in Obstetrics & Gynecology, 31*(2), 116–119. https://doi.org/10.1097/GCO.0000000000000524

Yonkers, K. A. (2007). The treatment of women suffering from depression who are either pregnant or breastfeeding. *American Journal of Psychiatry, 164*, 1457–1459.

Zanoli, P. (2004). Role of hyperforin in the pharmacological activities of St. John's wort. *CNS, 10*, 203–218.

Zhang, Y., Betran, A. P., Li, X., Liu, D., Yuan, N., & Shang, L. (2022). What is an appropriate caesarean delivery rate for China: A multicentre survey. *British Journal of Obstetrics & Gynaecology, 129*(1), 138–147. https://doi.org/10.1111/1471-0528.16951

Zhang, Y., Mu, Y., Li, X., Sun, C., Ma, X., Li, S., Li, L., Zhang, Z., & Qi, S. (2022). Improved interhemispheric functional connectivity in postpartum depression disorder: Associations with individual target-transcranial magnetic stimulation treatment effects. *Frontiers in Psychiatry, 13*. https://doi.org/10.3389/fpsyt.2022.859453

Zhao, Y., Kane, I., Wang, J., Shen, B., Luo, J., & Shi, S. (2015). Combined use of the Postpartum Depression Screening Scale (PDSS) and Edinburgh Postnatal Depression Scale (EPDS) to identify antenatal depression among Chinese pregnant women with obstetric complications. *Psychiatry Research, 226*, 113–119.

Zhou, C., Tabb, M. M., Sadatrafiei, A., Grun, F., Sun, A., & Blumberg, B. (2004). *Journal of Clinical Immunology, 24*, 623–636.

Zlotnick, C., Miller, I. W., Pearlstein, T., Howard, M., & Sweeney, P. (2006). A preventive intervention for pregnant women on public assistance at risk for postpartum depression. *American Journal of Psychiatry, 163*, 1443–1445.

Zlotnick, C., Tzilos, G. K., Miller, I. W., Seifer, R., & Stout, R. (2016). Randomized controlled trial to prevent postpartum depression in mothers on public assistance. *Journal of Affective Disorders, 189*, 263–268.

Index

AAP *see* American Academy of Pediatrics
abuse, sexual 98
ACOG screening guidelines 7
activity 57–59, 66
acupuncture: and antidepressants 66; and
    Chinese herbal medicine 66; groups 65;
    sham 65
acute phase 51, 99
adolescent maternity program 16
adult primary care 78
affective disorders 40, 43
age 7, 41, 44, 49, 59, 62, 76, 96, 100
ALA (alpha-linolenic acid) 38–39, 42
alpha-linolenic acid *see* ALA
American Academy of Pediatrics (AAP) 5, 9, 20
American College of Obstetricians and
    Gynecologists 7, 20
American mothers 14, 19
amino acid 37; proinflammatory 48
amygdala 66–67
anesthesia 65–66, 68

antenatal 16; education program 84; *see also*
    prenatal
anticoagulants 52
anticonvulsants 52
antidepressants 7, 27, 30, 35–36, 41, 47,
    50–54, 61, 64, 66, 67–68, 95–96;
    botanical 47; prescribed 98; refused 61;
    standard 50–52
antidepressant studies 52, 62
anti-HIV treatments 52
anti-inflammatory 59; effects 51, 95; of
    cognitive therapy 95
anxiety 4, 7, 9, 13, 15–17, 19, 21–22, 25–26,
    39–40, 43, 48–49, 57–58, 71–72, 80,
    83, 85, 91–95; generalized 21, 95;
    measures 16, 21; and PTSD 91; trait 49
anxiety scale 22; subscale 16, 25
ARA (arachidonic acid) 38
arachidonic acid 38–39, 42; proinflammatory 49
arachidonic acid cascade 41
Australia 13, 21, 38, 41–43, 48, 92
Ayers, S. 24–25

B-12 37, 47–49, 53; deficiencies 47, 53; levels
    49; lowest 49
barriers 4–8, 56–58, 78; addressing 7; to
    care 6, 78; mothers overcame 58; to
    screening 4, 6; significant 4
Beck, C. T. 23–24
Beck Depression Inventory 13, 23–24, 98
beliefs 4, 28, 96; distorted 92; dysfunctional
    92; negative 93
benefits 5, 44, 57–59, 99
bias 57, 85
bipolar disorder 9, 23, 27, 29, 40–41, 52, 63,
    68; relapse 27
bipolar II 27
birth 17, 21, 24–26, 43, 61, 72, 77, 82,
    84–85, 87
birth trauma symptoms 25–26
birthweight 44
black cohosh 52
Black women 4, 16
BMI (body mass index) 48–49, 96
bonding: disordered 86; impaired 93; normal
    86; promoted 84
brain 39, 42, 65–68, 71, 74, 91–92, 96; activity
    67, 71; function 66; regions 66, 71
breast 82
breastfeeding 29, 36, 45, 47, 52–53, 59–60,
    73, 79, 82, 84, 94, 96, 98; babies 44;
    cessation 5; duration 73 (decreased 59);
    goals 73; increasing 79; initiation 6, 73;
    practices 67; problems 94 (self-reported
    94); rates 81; self-efficacy 85; studies
    44; support 73; woman 68
breastmilk samples 53
bright light and exercise 64
bright light therapy 36, 61–64
British mothers 57

caffeine 26–27
calcium, releasing 48; absorption, intestinal 47;
    imbalance 48
CAM (complementary and alternative)
    therapies 36

Canada 4–5, 93
Canadian new mothers 15, 71
cardiovascular disease 47–48, 96
caregiving 59, 83
Center for Epidemiologic Studies-Depression 11, 13, 20
Center for Epidemiologic Studies-Depression Scale 13
cerebellum: mediating 71; right 72
cesareans 7
child 5–6, 9, 20, 43, 68, 79
child abuse 81, 98
child allergy 40
childcare 58, 72, 76
childhood sexual abuse *see* CSA
child maltreatment 5
child neurodevelopment 40
child program 84
child relationships 5
children 43–44, 84–85
chilla 77
China 39, 80
Chinese 24, 94–95
Chinese herbal medicine 66
Chinese practice of confining women 48
circadian rhythms 63–64; desynchronizes 62
clinic, inner-city well-child 20
clinical interview, structured 14–15, 20, 72
clinical takeaways 8, 11, 18, 22, 27, 31, 37, 60, 64, 68, 74, 80, 96, 100
clinical trials: controlled 52; randomized 40
Clinician-Administered PTSD Scale 26
clinicians 5, 13, 20, 22, 29, 35, 41, 55, 64, 79, 98
cod-liver oil 44
cognitive-behavioral therapy 72, 80, 91–93, 95–96; and interpersonal psychotherapy 72, 91, 93
cognitive impairment 23
cognitive processing therapy *see* CPT
cognitive therapies for postpartum depression 92, 97
communities 4–6, 10, 18, 22, 30, 35–37, 68, 80, 83
community: interventions 69, 72–86; organizations 28; resources 8; services 79; settings 11; support 71, 75, 78, 80
comorbid conditions 4, 6, 8, 10, 14–26, 29–30
compassion 76, 95
complementary and integrative treatments 36, 40–68
compulsions 30
concentration, impaired 23, 61
consciousness 93
contact 30, 78–79, 83; skin-to-skin 82, 86
cortisol 60, 82; lower salivary 82
costs 36–37, 75, 78

counseling 4, 78, 92, 98
couples, high-hostility 96
COVID-19 pandemic 21, 43, 49, 72, 78
COX enzymes 49
CPT 104–105
C-reactive protein 49, 96; lowered 96
CSA 102
cultural: adaptation 14; background 22; differences 78; identity 76
cultures 14–15, 35, 71, 76–77, 79
curcumin 37, 47, 49, 53–54
curcuminoid 49
cytokines 51, 96; anti-inflammatory 42; circulating 60; inflammatory 47

DASS-21 (Depression and Anxiety Scale) 25–26
dawn simulation 61, 63
delivery 40, 44–45, 54, 82, 99
demographic factors 26, 48, 76
Denmark 83
Dennis, C.-L. 11, 14–15, 78
depressed: adolescents, low-income 98; mood 20, 55; mothers 5–6, 18, 24, 29, 60, 71, 84, 99; women, pregnant 94
depression 4–30, 35–36, 38–43, 45–51, 53–68, 71–74, 78–87, 91–100; alleviated 61; assessed 21, 57, 84; care management 79 (telephone-delivered 79); centers 67; comorbid 9; education 79; and hostility 96; identifying 4, 9, 16, 20; items 21; lower 41, 57, 63, 66–67, 77, 82; measured 21, 40, 48, 67; mild 6, 55, 72; minor 24; missed 13–14; non-seasonal 61; in partners 17; in pregnant women 24; prevalence, estimate 15; and PTSD 65; questions 20; rates 72, 83; reducing 57, 91; resources 84; risk 71–73; scores 66, 95; and support 99; and trauma 72; treating 40–42, 55, 61, 67, 78, 91; treatments 57
depression and anxiety levels 67, 80
Depression and Anxiety Scale 22
depressive mood 16
depressive symptoms: decreased 58; lowered total 49; lowering 50; persistent 99; reduced 82, 92, 98–99; severe 18
depressive symptoms and lower use of medication 4
development: cognitive 43; fetal 96; vision 42
DHA (docosahexaenoic acid) 38–39; concentrations in breastmilk 45; consumption 40, 43; group 41; levels 44–45 (erythrocyte 43); supplementation 43

diabetes 47, 96; ameliorated 49; gestational
4, 57
diabetes mellitus 57
diagnostic criteria for postpartum depression 14
digital self-help/support 75, 78, 80
discriminant validity 26
dopamine 39
dosages 41, 44, 50–53
DSM-5 14–15, 25; criteria for posttraumatic
stress disorder 24–26

eating disturbances 23
ECT 66, 68
eczema 44
Edinburgh Postnatal Depression Scale 2–3, 13,
16, 23; US version 17; *see also* EPDS
education 7, 14, 20, 56, 79, 81, 83–87, 98;
education interventions 83, 86
effects 40, 49, 52–53, 56, 59, 67, 71–72, 78,
82, 84–85, 95, 99; of exercise 55–56,
59; of interpersonal psychotherapy
(IPT) 97, 99; of postpartum depression
7; therapeutic 40, 64, 91
eicosapentaenoic acid 38–39; *see also* EPA
electrical stimulation, mild 65
Emerging CAM Treatments 65, 67
emotional debt 95
emotional lability 23
emotional reactivity 94
emotional response 94
endocannabinoid system 42
endocrine disruptors 49
EPA 3, 38; and ARA in cell membranes 38;
and DHA supplements 41–43
EPA/DHA 39–42, 44
EPDS: EPDS-2 16; EPDS-3 12, 16, 18, 21;
EPDS and PHQ 13, 27; EPDS and
PHQ-9 13, 27; EPDS-Lifetime 17;
EPDS-Partners 17; EPDS scores 17, 24,
29, 62, 67, 84, 95; EPDS-US 12, 17–18;
for prenatal screening 16; *see also*
Edinburgh Postnatal Depression Scale
Epidemiologic Studies Depression Scale 11,
13, 20
equity 4, 75–76
erythrocytes 45
Europe 26, 39
evidence 5, 37, 40, 43, 45, 47, 51, 66–67, 95
exercise: aerobic 55, 57–59; at-home 60;
exercise interventions 56–57, 60; for
milder depressions 55; moderate-
intensity 57–58; supervised 55–56, 58;
type 58

false negatives 10–11
families 5, 28, 30, 71–72, 74, 76, 80; minority
98; new 87

family: dysfunction 5; health 5, 9, 20; history
29; members 4, 28, 75
Faroe Islands 44
fathers 17, 25, 73
fatigue 26, 58, 61–62
fatty acids 36–39, 40–42, 45, 59
fear 4, 23–25, 30
feeding method 26
fish consumption 39, 44;
population-level 39
fish intake 40, 44
fish oil 46
fish oil capsules 38, 45
fluoxetine 51
fMRI 66, 72
forgiveness 95
Freeman, M. P. 5, 36, 38, 40, 44
functional connectivity strength 71–72

GABAergic activity 51
Gable, R. K. 23
GAD-2 21
galactagogue 49
gamma linoleic acid 39
general anxiety disorders 7 21
Generalized Anxiety Disorder-2 Scale 21
general practitioners (GPs) 7
gestation 39–40, 43–45, 48, 57
goal 13, 15, 17, 23, 75, 79, 92, 97, 99
GPs 7; *see also* general practitioners
gray matter volume 66
Great Britain 50
groups 7, 10, 13, 20, 23, 50–51, 55–60, 62,
65, 67, 71–72, 79, 82–85, 91–93, 95,
98–100; comparison 49, 57; control
(standard-care 56, 78; usual-care 83,
95; wait-list 83, 93, 98); exercise/
education 56; exercise/medication
55; high-risk 85; infant-massage 85;
medication/exercise 55; skin-to-skin 82
group sessions/support 71, 77, 83, 99–100
guilt 58
gynecologists 7, 20

Hamilton Depression Rating Scale 13, 20, 41,
50, 58, 62, 65–66, 98
harm 15, 23, 28–30, 45, 73
health 5, 21, 38, 93, 96; maternal/child 79;
problems 85, 93
healthcare 36, 79
healthcare providers 4, 11–12, 18, 27, 52–54,
58, 71, 75, 77, 79–81, 97; settings 4,
20; support 75, 77, 79
health organizations 19, 65
health-related quality of life 58, 62
health system 8, 76
heart disease 59

heart rate 42
helplessness 24–25
herbal antidepressant 50, 52, 54
Hibbeln, J. R. 39
hippocampal neurogenesis 42
Hispanics 72, 98, 100
home visiting 81; education 81, 83, 85, 87; and infant massage 81
home visitors 81–82
homocysteine 48–49
Hong Kong 39
hopelessness 20, 29
horror 24–25
hospital-grade pump 29
hospitalization 28–29
hostility 60, 95–96
HPA axis 49
Humphrey, S. 52
husband 30, 73–74
hyperactivation 64
hyperarousal 24–25
hyperforin 50–53
hyperglycemia 47
hypericin 50, 52–53
Hypericum Depression Trial Study Group 50
hypericum perforatum 50; *see also* St. John's wort
hyperinsulinemia 47
hyperparathyroidism 48
hypertension 44, 57; developing 44; gestational 57; persistent pulmonary 93; pregnancy-associated 4
hypothalamus 63

ICD-10 (International Classification of Diseases-10) 14–15
Iceland 44
IL-1α (interleukin-1-alpha) 96
IL-1β (interleukin-1-beta) 42, 49, 51, 96
IL-2 (interleukin-2) 51
IL-6 (interleukin-6); decreased 96; elevated 43, 96
IL-8 (interleukin-8) 96
IL-10 (interleukin-10) 42
imipramine 50
immune-inflammatory system 64
immune system 44, 96
immunization clinics 5
infant attachment 85–86; care 84; coaching 86; dose, relative 53; dyads 86; exposure 53; massage 84–86; mortality 43; plasma 53; safety 30; salivary oxytocin pre 86; weight 53
infants 5–6, 23, 25–26, 28, 30, 44, 52–53, 58–59, 68, 78, 81–87, 92

infections 29, 96
inflammation, systemic 60; and anxiety 40; levels 38
inflammatory: diseases 47, 49; marker 51; response systems 42, 49
informal community settings interventions 71
inner-city women 57
insomnia 27, 29, 64
insula 67
insulin receptor signal transduction 47
integrative treatment for perinatal depression 33, 35–37, 40–68
interhemispheric communication 67
interpersonal: conflicts 97; deficits 97; disputes 97
interpersonal psychotherapy 72, 91, 97–100
intervention 9, 18, 48, 57–58, 71–72, 75–80, 82–84, 86, 92–93, 95, 97–100; mindfulness-based 95
intervention mothers 84
Iran 85
Italy 40

Japan 39–40, 42–43

kava 52
Kendall-Tackett, K. A. 42
Kenya 20
key findings 9, 12, 19, 23, 28, 35, 38, 55, 61, 65, 71, 75, 81, 91
Kiecolt-Glaser, J. K. 38, 42, 59–60, 95–96
Kim, J. J. 7
Kim, Y.-D. 65
Kroenke, K. 19, 21

labor 76, 84
lactation 43–44, 48, 53, 75–76
lactic acid 59
LactMed 50, 52
life stresses 55, 72, 94
lifetime adversities 72
lifetime incidence of postpartum depression 17
light 62–64; bright 61–64; intensity 62; lower-intensity 61–63; output 64; receptors 64; red 62; therapy 61, 64; visor 62
light boxes 61–64
linoleic acid 39
LMIC (low- and middle-income countries) 14, 77
low-income women 20, 76

Maes, M. 42
major depression 9–11, 13, 15, 17, 19, 21, 23–24, 27–28, 41, 44, 50–51, 53, 55–56, 62–63, 65, 92, 96, 98; history of 17, 98; treating 67–68

males 86
MAOIs 115, 116, 118, 120
MARS (Mobile App Rating Scale) 80
massage group 65, 84–85
mastitis 29
maternal mood 82
Maternal Social Support Index (MSSI) 74
maternal suicide risk 28
maternal warmth 95
MBCT (mindfulness-based cognitive therapy) 93–95
MDQ *see* Mood Disorder Questionnaire
measure postpartum feelings 23
measures: birth trauma 24; of depression and anxiety 21; of PTSD 21; sleep problems 23
MedEdPPD 6
medical emergencies 25–26
medications: for depressed low-income adolescents 98; and psychotherapy 35, 51; in randomized trials 55; in treating depression 91, 97
medicinal plant 50
melatonin 63–64
mental health 5–7, 18, 39, 47, 56, 60, 66, 76, 78, 81–82, 85–86, 96; disorders 7, 14; practices 82; practitioners 8, 79; support 82
metabolic syndrome 96
metabolism 39, 47, 52, 59
metabolite 37
midwives 7–8, 23, 76, 78, 82
migrants 72
mindfulness-based cognitive therapy *see* MBCT
mindfulness in intervention studies 94–95
Misri, S. 92
Mobile App Rating Scale (MARS) 80
monoamine oxidase inhibitors *see* MAOIs
monotreatment 41, 68, 92
Mood Disorder Questionnaire (MDQ) 27
morning light exposure 61, 63–64
Moses-Kolko, E. L. 28
mothers 4–12, 14–18, 20–21, 25–31, 35, 37, 40–47, 49, 52–56, 58–64, 68, 71, 73, 75–87, 92–95, 97–99; anxious 92; disadvantaged 72; first-time 83; low-education 20; lower-income 5; non-depressed 24
mothers and: babies 45; families 76; fathers 73; volunteers 77
motivational interviewing 84
MSPSS (Multidimensional Scale of Perceived Social Support) 74
MSSI (Maternal Social Support Index) 74
Multidimensional Scale of Perceived Social Support (MSPSS) 74

NAMI (National Alliance on Mental Illness) 61, 63–64
National Network of Depression Centers 67
natural killer cell cytotoxicity 96
neonatal adaptation 93
Neonatal Behavioral Assessment Scale 82
neonatal intensive care unit *see* NICU
neuropeptide 49
neurotransmitters 39, 51
new mothers 4, 6–7, 9–10, 12, 20, 23, 25, 58–59, 61, 63, 71, 73, 77, 80–81, 83, 91
New Zealand 38
NICU (neonatal intensive care unit) 26, 62, 85
non-depressed women 17, 40, 48
non-pharmacologic treatments 6, 36, 95
norepinephrine 39
Norway 39, 43
nurses 76, 83
nutraceuticals 37–39, 41, 43, 45, 47, 49, 51, 53

obsessive-compulsive disorder (OCD) 30, 67, 91, 93; thoughts 28
obstetrician-gynecologist 7–8, 20, 23
OCD *see* obsessive-compulsive disorder
O'Hara 7, 76, 92–93, 98
Oman 49
omega-3s 38–46; anti-inflammatory 38; long-chain 36–38; low 40; parent 38; recommended 40
omega-6s 38–41; and omega-3s 38–39
oxytocin 81–82, 84, 86; receptors 81, 84; response 86

pain 49, 60, 67, 94; chronic 65–66, 91
pandemic 72
Pandora's box 4–5, 8
panic attacks 29
panic disorder 16–17, 21, 30, 93
paraprofessionals 100
parathyroid 48
parenting stress 17, 85, 92, 95
partners 17, 25, 71–73, 80, 83, 98–99; non-depressed 99
partners in treatment 99
patient education materials 82
Patient Health Questionnaire-2 8–9, 16, 20
Patient Health Questionnaire-4 4, 21
Patient Health Questionnaire-9 9, 19–21
PCL-5 (PTSD Checklist-5) 25–26
pediatricians 5–8; screening for postpartum depression 6
pediatrics 5
peers 75–79, 81, 93
peer support 75, 83; and healthcare providers 75; in-person 78; tried online 80

Perceived Stress Scale 60
perceived support 71, 74
perinatal: anxiety disorders 16; depression 5,
    21, 39–41, 53, 58, 61, 64, 72; period
    7, 10, 26, 42, 71, 79; women 7, 10, 19,
    23, 26, 40, 43, 47, 57, 62, 65, 68, 91,
    93, 97
pharmacokinetics 53
pharmacotherapy 27
physical activity 56–60
physicians 6, 57
physiological downregulation 91
Pilates program 58
pineal gland 63–64
placebo effect 41–42, 50, 67
plasma 41–42, 52–53, 60
plasma norepinephrine 42
Portugal 24
postpartum 7–9, 15–17, 21–22, 27, 39–40,
    44, 55–56, 58, 67–68, 74, 76, 78–79,
    82, 84, 91–95, 97–100
postpartum adjustment 84, 99; and social
    support 99
Postpartum Bonding Questionnaire 86
postpartum depression: in adolescents 72–73;
    ameliorating 86; experienced 76;
    in high-risk women 99; lifetime 17;
    possible 48; prevented 92; in teens 73;
    treated 78, 97
postpartum depression forum 80
postpartum education 73
postpartum period 12, 23, 27, 58; early 12
postpartum psychosis 27, 29
postpartum support 75, 80
Postpartum Support International (PSI) 79
postpartum women, healthy 66
posttraumatic stress disorder 21, 26;
    see also PTSD
practitioners 8, 23, 35–36, 55, 65, 71
predisposition 36
preeclampsia 57
prefrontal cortex: dorsolateral 68; left
    dorsolateral 67; left ventrolateral 72
pregnancy 4, 7, 9, 17, 20–21, 27, 30, 40–46,
    53, 55–57, 62, 64, 83, 91–93, 95, 97,
    99–100; complications 24
Pregnancy Risk Assessment Monitoring
    Systems 8, 20
pregnant women, low-income 98–99
prematurity 93
prenatal 18, 73, 76, 83; anxiety 57; clinics
    14; depression 48, 58, 77; exercise 58;
    exposure 49; screening 16; stress 43
preprohormone 47
Preston, J. 26, 36
preterm birth 4, 25, 38, 40, 43, 45–46
preterm infants 85, 93

preventing depression 99
primary care 4, 19, 78–79, 98; pediatric 78
primary care healthcare providers 5–6
primary care sample 19
programs 11, 18, 27, 56, 72, 75–87, 94–96
proinflammatory cytokines 42–43, 45, 49, 51,
    59–60, 64, 96; IL-1α 42; IL-1β 59
prolactin 52
prospective cohort studies 48
providers 4, 6–8, 26, 36, 68, 78–79, 81
PSI (Postpartum Support International) 79
psychiatric illness 45
psychiatrists 7, 98
psychometric properties 21, 26
psychosis 30
psychosocial 5, 9, 20, 29, 56
psychotherapy 35–37, 51, 56, 68, 71–72, 86,
    89–100
PTSD: birth-related 24; diagnosis 25–26;
    PTSD Checklist-5 25

racial/ethnic minorities 21, 76
randomization 78, 85
randomized controlled trials (RCTs.) 40–41,
    43–44, 48, 50–51, 55–58, 62, 65,
    67–68, 79–80, 82, 85, 91, 94–95
recovery 48, 55, 74, 76, 85, 97–99
referrals 5–6, 11, 18, 30, 78
refugees 72
relationships 48, 56, 59, 71, 77, 96–97, 99;
    establishing close 96; key 97; marital 92;
    mother's 92; personal 99; unstable 98
relationship status 76
relaxation 93
reliability, good 18–19, 22, 24–26
reliability and validity 9–10, 12, 17, 21–22,
    24, 26
remission: achieved 67, 99; prolonged
    clinical 97
remission rates, higher 63
repetitive transcranial magnetic stimulation
    (rTMS) 65–68
resilience 42, 91, 94; increased 72
resources 4–6, 11, 27, 35, 75, 81, 83–84
responsiveness 73
risk 4–5, 28–30, 40, 42–45, 47–48, 53–55,
    57–58, 62–63, 71–74, 81, 83–84,
    87, 93, 96; for breastfeeding cessation
    5; for harming 28, 30; higher 20, 47;
    lower women's 81, 84; minimal 53; for
    postpartum depression 17; reducing 82
risk factors 17, 29, 96; modifiable 84;
    severe 98

safety 36, 43, 49, 51–53, 67, 93
SCID (Structured Clinical Interview for DSM)
    15, 20, 23, 98

scoring: errors 13; issues 12; mistakes 18; reverse 13; traditional 27
Scotland 18
screen: for anxiety and depression 21–23; for risk of maternal suicide 28
screening: for co-occurring anxiety and PTSD 9; for depression and comorbid conditions 4, 6, 8, 10, 12, 14–26, 30; for depression in pregnancy 12; goals 9, 11; in health settings 8; mandated depression 8, 82; in obstetric settings 7; in pediatric settings 5; and referral to community resources 5, 8; tools 12–13, 19, 21, 23–25, 27, 78
seasonal affective disorder 61, 63–64
selective-serotonin reuptake inhibitors (SSRIs) 51, 93
self-blame 16
self-care 6, 77
self-compassion 91, 94–95; Self-Compassion Scale 94
self-criticism 58
self-efficacy 57, 73, 95
self-esteem 83, 85, 94
self-harm/suicide 15
self-help 80
self-isolation 58
self-judgment 94
self-kindness 91, 94
self-reassurance 30
self-reports 17
sensitivity 9–10, 14–16, 19–21, 24–25, 27, 64
serotonin syndrome 52
sertraline 50–51, 55, 92
services 6, 75–78, 80–81
sessions 55, 59, 65, 67, 83–84, 92–93, 95, 98–99
severity 19, 25, 28, 58
sexual abuse survivors 79
sham treatments 68
Shetland Islands 44
side effects 36–37, 51–53, 62, 66, 98; benign 51, 68; toxic 51
Singapore 40
skin to skin 82
sleep 6, 17, 23, 26–27, 29–30, 62–63, 93, 96; difficulties 27, 86, 93, 96; parameters 93; in pregnant women 26; problems 17, 93; quality 48, 62; and social support 93
social integration 71
social networks 99
social support 36–37, 60, 71–75, 78, 83–84, 93, 99
socioeconomic status 76, 82
South Africa 16, 39, 82
South Australia 95

Spain 25, 95
spouses 30, 92
standard care 49, 56, 78, 92, 99
St. John's wort, taking 47, 50, 52, 54
stress 26, 42, 49, 60, 84–85, 92–93, 98; high 60, 83; lower 60, 85, 92; oxidative 49; response 42, 81, 87; severe 30; symptoms 95; system 42, 91
Stress Scale-21 25–26
Structured Clinical Interview-Depression 15, 23, 98
Suarez, E. C. 96
substance abuse 28–29, 85
suicidal ideations 5, 11, 19, 24, 29, 41
suicide 28–29, 41; maternal 28–29; plans 28–29; risk 28–29, 41
sun 19, 47
support: affirmational 76; baseline 31, 77; building 97; continuous 78; emotional 76, 80, 82; empathetic 76, 78; family 72; functional 74; informational 71; in-person 78; instrumental 72, 80; low 73; new mother 78, 81; perceived social 72, 77; professional 75, 77; received 72, 83; relationship-based 83; responsive 71; sustained social 74
support for: breastfeeding 73; group 85; mothers 73, 78; for new mothers 81
suprachiasmatic nucleus 63
symptoms 4, 9, 15, 19, 24–25, 27–31, 35–37, 49, 52, 58, 61–66, 92, 96, 98; arousal-related 49; birth-related 25; common 18; general 25; milder 9; monitor 26; monitoring 79; psychophysiological 42; psychotic 30; severe 13–15, 28; somatic 18; suicide risk, possible infant harm 29, 31
systematic review 30, 36, 48, 97

Taiwan 39, 58
task-based support 71, 74
tDCS (transcranial direct current stimulation) 65–68
teens 73, 98
telephone support: one-on-one 77–79
teratogenic effects 44; possible 36
therapists 92, 97–98
thinking: delusional 30; negative 94; obsessive 23
thoughts 6–7, 28, 30, 71, 74, 84, 91–92, 94; of infant harm 28, 30; suicidal 24
Traditional Chinese Medicine 66, 68
training 5–6, 8, 75–76, 94
transcranial direct current stimulation (tDCS) 65–68
translations 14, 19
trauma 24–25, 42, 72

treatment 5–6, 8, 11, 35–37, 40, 47, 49–51,
    53–58, 60–63, 65–68, 83–85, 87,
    91–93, 95–99; algorithms 6; choices
    35, 55, 64; conditions 63, 79; effects,
    largest 98; for partners 99; protocol 80;
    for PTSD 93; team 76
turmeric, spice 49

universal screening 4, 7–8
US National Center for PTSD 26
US Pharmacopeia 45, 52
USPSTF (US Preventive Services Task Force) 4,
    7, 9–10
usual care 4, 82, 84–85, 98–99

validity 9–10, 12, 16–19, 21–22, 24–26
vitamin: B-12 47–48, 53; D 47–48
volunteers 76–79

Wang, C. 39
Wang, J. 67
Wang, Y. 108
Wang, Y. 48
well-baby 5, 16, 20
Wisner, K. L. 6, 27, 79
women 4–7, 10, 14–17, 20–21,
    24–27, 29–30, 36, 39–45,
    47–49, 52–60, 62–63, 66–67,
    71–74, 77–79, 82–83, 92, 94,
    96–100; examined 71;
    helping 86; lower-income 76;
    migrant 72; premenopausal 96;
    treated 66
work 37, 42, 50, 68, 72, 76–78, 97

Yoga 56, 58; examined 58; gentle 94
yoga group 58

Printed in the United States
by Baker & Taylor Publisher Services